TELL YOUR CHILDREN

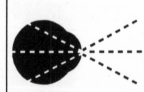

This Large Print Book carries the
Seal of Approval of N.A.V.H.

TELL YOUR CHILDREN

THE TRUTH ABOUT MARIJUANA, MENTAL ILLNESS, AND VIOLENCE

ALEX BERENSON

THORNDIKE PRESS
A part of Gale, a Cengage Company

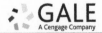

Farmington Hills, Mich • San Francisco • New York • Waterville, Maine
Meriden, Conn • Mason, Ohio • Chicago

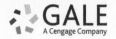

Copyright © 2019 by Alex Berenson.
Thorndike Press, a part of Gale, a Cengage Company.

ALL RIGHTS RESERVED
Thorndike Press® Large Print Lifestyles.
The text of this Large Print edition is unabridged.
Other aspects of the book may vary from the original edition.
Set in 16 pt. Plantin.

> **LIBRARY OF CONGRESS CIP DATA ON FILE.**
> **CATALOGUING IN PUBLICATION FOR THIS BOOK**
> **IS AVAILABLE FROM THE LIBRARY OF CONGRESS**
>
> ISBN-13: 978-1-4328-6041-7 (hardcover)

Published in 2019 by arrangement with Free Press, an imprint of Simon & Schuster, Inc.

Printed in Mexico
1 2 3 4 5 6 7 2 32 22 12 01 9

For Lucy and Ezra

The loveliest trick of the Devil is to persuade you that he does not exist.

> — C. P. Baudelaire,
> "The Generous Gambler"

CONTENTS

PART THREE: THE RED TIDE

INTRODUCTION: EVERYTHING YOU'RE ABOUT TO READ IS TRUE

In the early morning hours of December 19, 2014, in Cairns, Australia, a subtropical city of 160,000, Raina Thaiday stabbed eight children to death.

Seven of the kids were hers. The eighth was her niece. She was 37 years old. And she was very, very sick.

The case was among the worst incidents of maternal child killing ever recorded. But Cairns is a long way from anywhere, and Thaiday was the opposite of a glamorous defendant, a poor single mother. Within a month, she and her children had largely been forgotten. The house they haunted would be torn down, its grounds turned into a memorial.

So neither the killing nor the ultimate verdict in Thaiday's case attracted much interest.

They should have. They are signal events, proof of hidden horrors present and worse

11

to come.

On April 6, 2017, before about twenty spectators in Brisbane, Australia's third-largest city, Justice Jean Dalton of the Supreme Court of Queensland heard testimony from Thaiday's psychiatrists. A month later, Dalton released her finding.

"Ms. Thaiday had a mental illness," Dalton wrote. "She is entitled to the defence of unsoundness of mind. There is just no doubt." Thaiday had broken from reality when she killed her kids, Dalton wrote. She couldn't control her actions. In medical terms, she suffered from psychosis and the devastating mental illness schizophrenia, which can cause hallucinations, delusions, and paranoia.

Nearly 1 percent of people will be diagnosed with schizophrenia in their lives. Many more will have other types of psychosis. Schizophrenia, the most severe form, usually strikes in the late teens or twenties. The disorder has a strong genetic component; scientists estimate almost half of the risk comes from genetic factors. Men are diagnosed more often than women, and in the United States, black people more often than those of other races, though researchers are not sure why.

Some drugs help control its symptoms,

but schizophrenia has no cure. Most of its sufferers do not work, marry, or have families. They die on average about fifteen years younger than other Americans.

People with schizophrenia are also far more likely to commit violent crime. Mental illness advocacy groups play down that grim reality. "Most people with mental illness are not violent," the National Alliance on Mental Illness explains on its website. "In fact, people with mental illness are more likely to be the victims of violence."

Those statements are deeply misleading. They tuck schizophrenia into the broader category of "mental illness," including depression. In reality, men with a schizophrenia diagnosis are five times as likely to commit violent crimes as healthy people. For women, the gap is even greater.

"They're at an increased risk for crime, they're at a very increased risk for violent crime," says Dr. Sheilagh Hodgins, a professor at the University of Montreal who has studied mental illness and violence for more than thirty years. Hodgins acknowledges that discussing the issue can cause people with schizophrenia to be stigmatized. "The best way to deal with the stigma is to reduce the violence," she says.

Indeed, over the last century, societies

have recognized that people with severe mental illness cannot always be held responsible for their actions. Courts accept "not guilty by reason of insanity" as a valid defense, even for murder.

As insanity cases go, Thaiday's was uncontroversial. The psychiatrists who testified before Justice Dalton agreed she was psychotic when she killed her children. She was paranoid and delusional before the murders. She made no effort to flee afterward. She stabbed herself and then waited outside her house, talking to herself and God, until her son Lewis found her.

Thaiday's delusional thinking continued after she was hospitalized at "The Park" — a psychiatric hospital in Brisbane once known as the Woogaroo Lunatic Asylum. Despite medicine meant to help her control her thoughts, Thaiday fantasized about killing other patients.

Thus, Justice Dalton determined that when she murdered her kids, Thaiday "was suffering from a mental illness, paranoid schizophrenia, and that she had no capacity to know what she was doing was wrong." Had Dalton ended her verdict there, the case would have been just another awful story of untreated mental illness. But she didn't. She found Thaiday's illness was no accident.

Marijuana had caused it.

"Thaiday gave a history of the use of cannabis since she was in grade 9," Dalton wrote. "All the psychiatrists thought that it is likely that it is this long-term use of cannabis that caused the mental illness schizophrenia to emerge."

With those words, Dalton made one of the first judicial findings anywhere linking marijuana, schizophrenia, and violence — a connection that cannabis advocates are desperate to hide.

I know what a lot of you are thinking right now.

This is propaganda. Marijuana is safe. Way safer than alcohol. Barack Obama smoked it. Bill Clinton smoked it too, even if he didn't inhale. Might as well say it causes presidencies. I've smoked it myself, I liked it fine. Maybe I got a little paranoid, but it didn't last. Nobody ever died from smoking too much pot.

Yeah, this is silly. Reefer Madness, man!

I know you're thinking it, because it's what you've been told for the last twenty-five years. And because I once thought it, too. My wife, Jacqueline, is a psychiatrist who specializes in evaluating mentally ill criminals. If you commit a serious crime in the state of New York and claim an insanity defense, you may well talk to her. And one fine night a couple of years ago, we were talking about a case, the usual horror story, somebody who'd cut up his grandmother or set fire to his apartment — typical bedtime chat in the Berenson house — and she said something like, "Of course he was high, been smoking pot his whole life."

"Of course?" I said.

"Yeah, they all smoke."

"Well . . . other things too, right?"

"Sometimes. But they all smoke."

"So, marijuana causes schizophrenia?"

I'd smoked a few times in my life. I remember walking down an Amsterdam street in 1999, laughing uncontrollably, a twenty-something American cliché. I never took to the stuff, but I had no moral problem with it. If anything, I tended to be a libertarian on drugs, figuring people ought to be allowed to make their own mistakes. I'd watched the legalization votes in Colorado and elsewhere without much interest. Of course, I'd heard of *Reefer Madness,* the notorious 1936 movie that showed young people smoking marijuana and descending into insanity and violence. The film's lousy acting has turned it into unintentional satire, an easy way for advocates of legalization to mock anyone who claims cannabis might be dangerous.

I'm not sure if I said to my wife that night, Oh, please, but I thought it. Jacqueline would have been within her rights to say, I trained at Harvard and Columbia. Unlike you. I know what I'm talking about. Unlike you. Maybe quit mansplaining. Instead she offered something neutral like, I think that's what the big studies say. You should read them.

Hmm, I thought. Maybe I should read them.

People have smoked marijuana for thousands of years to feel the effects of delta-9-tetrahydrocannabinol, commonly called THC. The cannabis plant naturally produces the compound. Among other effects, THC can induce euphoria, enhance sensation, distort the perception of time, and increase hunger — the infamous munchies.

For most of the twentieth century, cannabis possession and use were illegal in the United States. The modern wave of legalization began in 1996, when stories of suffering AIDS patients moved California voters to approve cannabis use with a doctor's okay. By 2006, ten more states had allowed medical marijuana.

Now the wave has become a tsunami. In 2012, Colorado and Washington became the first states to approve recreational use. As of summer 2018, seven more states, including California and the District of Columbia, had joined them. In those states, anyone 21 or over can walk into a dispensary and buy "flower" — traditional smokable marijuana — as well as "edibles" such as THC-infused chocolate, and "wax" or "shatter," high-potency extracts that are nearly pure THC. In all, two hundred million Americans have gained access to medical or recreational marijuana in the last twenty years. More than 60 percent of Americans now support legalized cannabis, polls show.

Marijuana advocates are now targeting federal laws, the last bulwark against national legalization. They have every reason to believe they will succeed. "The broader question of whether marijuana is going to get legalized is not really an interesting question right now," says Ethan Nadelmann, who is probably more responsible for the legalization of cannabis in the United States than anyone else. "I don't think it's really stoppable."

Like Raina Thaiday's illness, the charge to legalization is no accident. It has come after a long, expensive, and shrewd lobbying effort that has been funded largely by a handful of the world's richest people. They have produced a sea change in public attitudes and policy in a shockingly short period — years, not generations.

The top lobbying groups have anodyne names like the Drug Policy Alliance and the Marijuana Policy Project. They argue that the real harm from cannabis comes from laws against it. Arrests leave young people with criminal records and damaged job prospects. Prohibition pushes trafficking and dealing on to a violent black market. Further, marijuana is a civil rights issue because police are more likely to arrest black and Hispanic people for smoking than whites.

But their goal is not marijuana decriminalization; it's legalization, a very different policy.

Many states have already decriminalized possession. Decriminalization puts marijuana in a twilight zone, neither legal nor illegal. Under decriminalization, police officers do not usually arrest people for carrying small amounts of marijuana. Instead they issue a ticket that carries a small fine and does not result in a criminal record.

Decriminalization sharply reduces the civil rights concerns that drug policy groups

19

raise. Arrests for marijuana possession fell by almost 90 percent in Massachusetts the year after that state decriminalized, for example. Even in states that haven't decriminalized, almost no one is imprisoned for possession anymore.

But though decriminalization protects users, growers and dealers still face criminal risk. Cannabis itself is still illegal and cannot be marketed. For the marijuana lobby, which now includes for-profit companies, decriminalization isn't a satisfactory compromise. Advocates want cannabis on equal footing with alcohol and tobacco. Full legalization makes cannabis a state-regulated drug that users can buy at retail dispensaries.

Across the country, advocates have followed the same playbook. They press for medical legalization, then argue for recreational use.

Linking legalization to medical use has proven the crucial step. It encourages voters to think of marijuana as something other than an intoxicant. In reality, except for a few narrow conditions such as cancer-related wasting, neither cannabis nor THC has ever been shown to work in randomized clinical trials. Such trials are the only reliable way to prove a drug works. The Food and Drug Administration requires them before prescription drug companies can sell new treatments.

But Americans are disillusioned with the FDA and those drug companies — for the prices they charge, the way they hide side effects, and now the scourge of prescription opioids. Cannabis backers present marijuana as a superior natural alternative. Amazon's digital shelves are filled with books such as *Marijuana Gateway to Health: How Cannabis Protects Us from Cancer and Alzheimer's Disease.* (Cannabis does work moderately as a pain reliever, though it is usually compared to a placebo rather than other pain relievers such as Advil or Tylenol, and a large Australian study recently cast doubt on its effectiveness in chronic pain.)

Further confusing the issue, one of the chemicals in marijuana, cannabidiol — usually called CBD — appears to have some medical benefits. But CBD is not psychoactive. Unlike THC, it doesn't get users high.

But many people don't understand the distinction between THC, CBD, and cannabis itself. Advocates have seized on the misunderstanding. They point to studies showing CBD's possible benefits to claim that marijuana has medical value. There's only one problem. Most cannabis consumed today — whether called "recreational" or "medical" — has lots of THC and almost no CBD, so whatever good CBD may do is irrelevant.

Yet the strategy has proven incredibly effective. Even though the FDA has never approved marijuana for any medical use, almost all Americans believe that "medical marijuana" should be legal. Even in states where medical marijuana is not legal, the constant drumbeat that marijuana is medicine has led people to believe the drug is safe and driven up consumption. In 2017, almost 10 percent of American teens and adults used marijuana at least once a month, a rise of more than 60 percent from a decade before. In states where marijuana is legal, rates are significantly higher. As many as one-third of young adults in states like Colorado are past-month users.

Those users tend to use heavily — much more heavily than the average drinker uses alcohol. Only 1 drinker in 15, or about 7 percent, drinks daily or almost daily. In comparison, about 20 percent of all cannabis users use at that rate, a percentage that has soared since 2005. That year, about three million Americans used cannabis daily or almost daily. By 2017, the number topped eight million, approaching the twelve million daily or near-daily drinkers. In other words, casual use of cannabis has risen only moderately in the last decade. But heavy use has soared — almost tripling.

All those people are using cannabis that by historical standards is shockingly potent. Through the mid-1970s, most marijuana consumed in the United States contained less than 2 percent THC. Today's users wouldn't even recognize that drug as marijuana. Marijuana sold at legal dispensaries now routinely contains 25 percent THC. Imagine drinking martinis instead of near-beer to get a sense of the difference in power. Wax and shatter aren't even cannabis at all; they are near-pure THC that's been extracted from the plant.

But the change in potency and consumption patterns has happened so quickly that it has gone largely unnoticed by nonusers. Drawing on their own experience, many older Americans naturally think of marijuana as a relatively weak drug that most people consume only occasionally in social settings such as concerts — when the reverse is now true.

Legalization advocates also tirelessly argue that marijuana is safer than other drugs. "There are no documented deaths due to marijuana," Gary Johnson, the libertarian candidate for president, said in August 2016.

Johnson is wrong.

It is true that dying of a marijuana overdose is practically impossible, while opiate and alcohol overdoses kill tens of thousands of Americans a year. But immediate toxicity is only one measure of dangerousness. Almost nobody dies from chain-smoking a pack of Marlboro Reds either. Still, tobacco causes more deaths than any other drug, mostly from cancer and heart disease.

Similarly, cannabis can be lethal in many ways. A study based on hospital admission data found that marijuana sharply increases the risk of heart attacks after smoking. Case reports back that finding. The risk of marijuana-impaired driving appears higher than previously understood, too. In states that have legalized recreational marijuana, fatal car accidents where the drivers have only THC in their blood and not alcohol or other drugs are soaring.

The Centers for Disease Control compiles information from all the death certificates in the United States; its database shows that more than 1,000 people who died between 1999 and 2016 had cannabis or cannabinoids — and no other drugs — listed on their certificates as a secondary cause of death by poisoning. (That is the traditional method of counting fatal overdoses.) The number soared from 8 in 1999 to 191 in 2016. British government statistics show a similar trend. There, 14 people died from overdoses related to cannabis alone between 2014 and 2016.

Those figures are a fraction of those who died from opiates. But they should put to rest the canard that marijuana has never killed anyone.

More recently, legalizers have argued marijuana can stem the opiate epidemic by weaning people off drugs like heroin. The theory cuts against generations of evidence — both anecdotal and scientific — that marijuana use often leads to the use of other drugs. In fact, the first efforts at marijuana legalization in the 1970s ended in part because cocaine use followed marijuana use sharply higher. Few serious researchers into drug addiction doubt this connection, though the reasons why remain hotly debated.

Yet the theory that marijuana can fix the opiate epidemic has become close to conventional wisdom since 2014, due largely to one paper that showed states that legalized medical marijuana before 2010 had a slower increase in opiate overdose deaths.

The finding is almost certainly misleading. More recent papers that incorporate post-2010 data show that opiate deaths are rising as fast or faster in states that have legalized medical cannabis. A New York University professor and I analyzed overdose and drug use data ourselves and found that states that had higher marijuana use had slightly more opiate deaths and significantly more cocaine use. Other recent studies that look at individuals over time — a much more powerful method of showing cause-and-effect than examining state-level data — also show a strong link between marijuana and opiate use.

The trend found in the 2014 paper probably results from geographic coincidence. The opiate epidemic started in Appalachia, while the first states to approve medical marijuana were in the West. Once states east of the Mississippi approved medical marijuana and the opiate epidemic spread the other way, the finding vanished.

Yet the more recent evidence has received almost no attention. Meanwhile, the 2014 paper — based on data that is now almost a decade old and has been proven wrong — continues to be quoted widely. And no one seems to have noticed that the United States and Canada, the two big Western countries that have by far the worst opioid epidemics, also have by far the highest rates of cannabis use.

The misinformation about marijuana and opiates is part of a much bigger issue. The marijuana lobby brands itself as young, hip, and diverse. Cannabis activists are woke, seeing through government propaganda. Never mind that scientists at the National Institute on Drug Abuse go out of their way these days to offer measured assessments of marijuana's risks and benefits.

The propaganda comes mostly from pro-cannabis groups.

Especially on the issue of cannabis and mental illness. The Drug Policy Alliance offers "10 Facts About Marijuana" on its website, including this question: "Does marijuana negatively impact mental health?"

Its answer: "There is no compelling evidence that marijuana causes some psychiatric disorders in otherwise healthy individuals . . . [T]hose with mental illness might actually be self-medicating with marijuana."

A reassuring answer, especially considering the DPA claims it promotes "policies that are grounded in science."

Too bad it's not true.

I am not a scientist or physician. But I covered the prescription drug industry for the *New York Times* for years. I learned how to read studies and research papers — and how to ask scientists about drug risks and side effects. Still, as I mentioned, when I began researching marijuana, mental health, and violence, I didn't expect much.

I was wrong.

On some level, what's strange is how obvious the link has been, and for how long. Hundreds of years before psychiatrists examined the intersection of brain and mind, before statisticians learned to tease out cause and effect, before chemists discovered THC, ordinary people all over Asia and the Middle East knew about cannabis. They viewed it like opium, a drug that offered euphoria — at a price. Opium and its derivatives caused users to become physically addicted and led to deadly overdoses. Cannabis produced insanity and violence.

The first comprehensive reference guide to herbs and drugs ever created, a Chinese pharmacopeia called the *Pen-ts'ao Ching,* warned that excessive cannabis smoking caused "seeing devils." By about 100 AD, Chinese physicians believed the drug "stimulate(d) uncontrollable violence and criminal inclinations," according to a botanist who wrote a 1974 paper on cannabis in China. In the Middle East and North Africa, people noted similar effects.

Almost two thousand years later, the evidence is still mounting. Dozens of well-designed studies have linked marijuana with psychosis and schizophrenia. Researchers have found marijuana users are much more likely to develop schizophrenia. People with the disease suffer more frequent and severe relapses if they smoke.

Even so, doctors and scientists have much to learn about the link between cannabis and mental illness. Most people will never have a psychotic episode while using marijuana. Some will have temporary breaks from reality. But an unlucky minority of users will develop full-blown schizophrenia. At this point, doctors have no way of predicting who they will be.

The long, complex, and diligent quest by scientists and psychiatrists to understand the link between marijuana and psychosis is a crucial part of what you are about to read. But — spoiler alert — the connection has been proven. Arguably the most important finding of all came in 2017, when the National Academy of Medicine issued a 468-page research report titled "The Health Effects of Cannabis and Cannabinoids."

Formerly called the Institute of Medicine, the academy is a nonprofit group that charters committees to examine scientific questions. Committee members serve as volunteers and are supposed to be unbiased and free of conflicts of interest. Their reports are the gold standard for scientific research and medical practice in the United States.

To produce the cannabis report, sixteen professors and doctors worked with a staff of thirteen for more than a year. It was the first time the academy had looked at the health effects of marijuana since 1999. The committee examined thousands of studies and papers and was careful not to overstate the evidence in either direction. For example, it reported that marijuana does not appear to cause lung cancer.

That's the good news. On mental health, the report is far grimmer. The committee found strong evidence that marijuana causes schizophrenia and some evidence that it worsens bipolar disorder and increases the risk of suicide, depression, and social anxiety disorder. "Cannabis use is likely to increase the risk of developing schizophrenia and other psychoses; the higher the use, the greater the risk," the scientists concluded.

The higher the use, the greater the risk. In

other words, marijuana in the United States has become increasingly dangerous to mental health in the last fifteen years, as millions more people consume higher-potency cannabis more frequently.

Yet cannabis advocates will not concede the issue. They argue cannabis use has risen since the 1960s, while psychosis has not. "Rates of schizophrenia and other psychiatric illnesses have remained flat even during periods of time when marijuana use rates have increased," the Drug Policy Alliance claims.

In reality, crucial and largely unnoticed data and research suggest otherwise.

Finding out how many Americans had a heart attack or were diagnosed with cancer last year is easy. The federal government compiles and publicizes those figures. Finding a similar count for schizophrenia or other severe mental illness is impossible. Not hard. Impossible. No one tracks psychotic disorders. Not the National Institute of Mental Health. Not the Centers for Disease Control. And not the states.

In Washington state, which until 2018 was the largest state to have legalized cannabis, not only does the health department not count schizophrenia, Dr. Cathy Wasserman

— the state epidemiologist for noninfectious conditions — says she doesn't see how it could.

"I do not believe we could develop valid and reliable statewide estimates," Wasserman says. Health laws strongly protect mental health information. Plus, no definite test for schizophrenia exists. No brain scan or blood sample confirms it. It's a "clinical" diagnosis. Doctors make it based on how someone is acting. Many people with schizophrenia are never diagnosed at all. They simply wind up in prison.

So maybe the rate of schizophrenia in the United States isn't increasing. But one important figure suggests it is. The number of people showing up at hospitals with psychosis has soared since 2006, alongside marijuana use.

Emergency rooms saw a 50 percent increase in the number of cases where someone received a primary diagnosis of a psychotic disorder between 2006 and 2014, the most recent year for which full data is available. By 2014, more than 2,000 Americans every day showed up or were brought to emergency rooms for schizophrenia and other psychoses — 810,000 people in all.

Worse, the number of emergency room visitors who were diagnosed primarily with psychosis and secondarily with problems with cannabis tripled over that period, from 30,000 to 90,000. By 2014, 11 percent of Americans who showed up in emergency rooms with a psychotic disorder also had a secondary diagnosis of marijuana misuse. (That figure has never previously been reported. It comes from an analysis of federal data that the NYU professor and I conducted.) It doesn't come close to including everyone who used marijuana, only those whose abuse or dependence was so severe that emergency room physicians could diagnose it. Most of those people had no other drug problems diagnosed, only marijuana.

Studies from Denmark and Finland — two countries where mental illness cases can be counted accurately on a national basis — have also shown recent increases in schizophrenia diagnoses, following rising cannabis use. But those studies have received almost no attention. And last fall, a 70,000-person federal survey showed skyrocketing rates of serious mental illness among young adults in the United States, the same people who are most likely to use cannabis. The survey showed that 2.6 million Americans aged 18 to 25 met the criteria for serious mental illness in 2017,

7.5 percent of all Americans in that age group. The percentage has doubled in the last decade. Older and younger Americans, who are less likely to use, have shown much smaller increases.

In fact, as the evidence has mounted, public attitudes toward marijuana safety have gone the other way. The confusion is easy to understand. Take cigarettes and cancer. Smoking causes the vast majority of lung cancers. Yet researchers and doctors needed decades to see the connection, decades more to prove it. Science is hard work.

The opioid crisis has also deflected attention from the new research. For health and law enforcement agencies, the effects of rising marijuana use are a slow-motion problem. The 70,000 annual drug overdose deaths are an immediate emergency.

"The size and scope of the opioid crisis has distracted people," says Dr. Nora Volkow, director of the National Institute on Drug Abuse. But the legalization lobby — and its supporters in the media — sure haven't helped.

In 2011, a 22-year-old named Jared Lee Loughner shot Congresswoman Gabrielle Giffords in Tucson, Arizona, wounding her and killing six other people. Loughner was mentally ill and had frequently smoked. But when a commentator named David Frum raised the potential link, he was roundly mocked. *The Atlantic* magazine called Frum's theory one of the "5 Strangest Explanations for Jared Loughner's Attack," along with suggestions that heavy metal songs might be responsible.

The reaction to Loughner's case is the rule, not the exception. Marijuana's advocates have the money, the cultural gatekeepers, and the elite media. The *Washington Post* — not *High Times,* the *Washington Post* — runs headlines such as "Marijuana May Be Even Safer Than Previously Thought, Researchers Say" and "11 Charts That Show Marijuana Has Truly Gone Mainstream."

Because everybody knows that if you smoke too much, you just eat Doritos until you fall asleep. Everybody knows *Reefer Madness* is a joke. Cops just want excuses to put black people in jail. And everybody knows marijuana should be legal.

The great villain in the story legalizers tell about prohibition is Harry Anslinger. Anslinger served as the head of the Federal Bureau of Narcotics — the predecessor of the modern Drug Enforcement Administration (DEA) — from 1930 to 1962. Anslinger once wrote that:

> Addicts may often develop delirious rage during which they are temporarily and violently insane . . . this insanity may take the form of a desire for self-destruction or a persecution complex to be satisfied only by the commission of some heinous crime.

The marijuana lobby views Anslinger as a racist anticannabis fanatic who exaggerated the drug's dangers to convince Congress to prohibit it.

They're partly right.

Anslinger was openly racist, and marijuana's association with immigrants from Mexico undoubtedly fueled the drive for prohibition.

Yet Mexico itself criminalized marijuana *seventeen years before* the United States, in 1920, after Mexican lawmakers became convinced the drug caused mental illness and violence. Were those law-makers motivated by anti-Hispanic prejudice too? Advocates for legalization have been too busy mocking Anslinger to wonder if he might be right.

Because the "delirious rage" he describes sounds a lot like psychosis. And the "heinous crime" he mentions is happening far more often than anyone understands. Raina Thaiday's case is exceptional only because she had so many victims.

If you were shaking your head before, you're really shaking it now, I imagine.

I don't blame you. Almost no one — not even the police officers who deal with it every day, not even most psychiatrists — publicly connects marijuana and crime. We all know alcohol causes violence, but somehow, we have grown to believe that marijuana does not, that centuries of experience were a myth. As a pediatrician wrote in a 2015 piece for the *New York Times* in which he argued that marijuana was safer for his teenage children than alcohol: "People who are high are not committing violence."

But they are. Almost unnoticed, the studies have piled up. On murderers in Pittsburgh, on psychiatric patients in Italy, on tourists in Spain, on emergency room patients in Michigan. Most weren't even designed to look for a connection between marijuana and violence, because no one thought one existed. Yet they found it.

In many cases, they have even found marijuana's tendency to cause violence is even greater than that of alcohol. A 2018 study of people with psychosis in Switzerland found that almost half of cannabis users became violent over a three-year period; their risk of violence was *four times* that of psychotic people who didn't use. (Alcohol didn't seem to increase violence in this group at all.)

The effect is not confined to people with preexisting psychosis. A 2012 study of 12,000 high school students across the United States showed that those who used cannabis were more than three times as likely to become violent as those who didn't, surpassing the risk of alcohol use. Even worse, studies of children who have died from abuse and neglect consistently show that the adults responsible for their deaths use marijuana far more frequently than alcohol or other drugs — and far, far more than the general population. Marijuana does not necessarily cause all those crimes, but the link is striking and large.

We shouldn't be surprised.

The violence that drinking causes is largely predictable. Alcohol intoxicates. It disinhibits users. It escalates conflict. It turns arguments into fights, fights into assaults, assaults into murders.

Marijuana is an intoxicant that can disinhibit users, too. And though it sends many people into a relaxed haze, it also frequently causes paranoia and psychosis. Sometimes those are short-term episodes in healthy people. Sometimes they are months-long spirals in people with schizophrenia or bipolar disorder.

And paranoia and psychosis cause violence. The psychiatrists who treated Raina Thaiday spoke of the terror *she* suffered, and they weren't exaggerating. Imagine voices no one else can hear screaming at you. Imagine fearing your food is poisoned or aliens have put a chip in your brain.

When that terror becomes too much, some people with psychosis snap. But when they break, they don't escalate in predictable ways. They take hammers to their families. They decide their friends are devils and shoot them. They push strangers in front of trains. The homeless man mumbling about God frightens us because we don't have to be experts on mental illness and violence to know instinctively that *untreated psychosis is dangerous.*

And finding violence and homicides connected to marijuana is all too easy.

Before legalization passed in states like Washington, advocates claimed that it might reduce crime. In the years since, politicians — and even some social scientists relying on very oddly constructed research — have claimed that violence *has* fallen in states that have legalized for recreational use. When he introduced a bill to legalize marijuana nationally in 2017, Cory Booker, a Democratic senator from New Jersey, said that those states "are seeing decreases in violent crime."

Booker is wrong. Completely.

All four of the states that legalized in 2014 and 2015 — Alaska, Colorado, Oregon, and Washington — have seen sharp increases in murders and aggravated assaults since legalization. Combined, the four states saw a 35 percent increase in murders and a 25 percent increase in assaults between 2013 and 2017, far outpacing the national trend, even after adjusting for changes in population. (Across the United States, murders have risen 20 percent and aggravated assaults 10 percent over that period.) Knowing exactly how many of these crimes are related to marijuana is impossible without researching each of them in detail, but police reports and arrest warrants show a clear connection in many cases.

In 2004, as a *New York Times* reporter, I investigated the electric stun guns known as Tasers. Taser International, their manufacturer, said they were "non-lethal." Yet people kept dying after being shocked. I talked to experts on electricity and the heart who said the shocks might kill.

Turned out Taser had done little research on the dangers of its weapons. Still, the company wouldn't acknowledge any risk. As far as I could tell, its logic went like this:

1. Tasers don't kill.
2. No one has ever died from being shocked.
3. Therefore, Tasers couldn't have killed this person either.
4. Therefore, Tasers don't kill.

Rinse and repeat.

Eventually, Taser had to bend to reality. Too many studies and autopsies raised the connection. The weapons now carry prominent warnings of their cardiac risks.

The people fighting to legalize marijuana believe as deeply in their cause as the brothers who ran Taser. In a 2013 interview with *Rolling Stone,* Ethan Nadelmann called prohibition an "absurdity" and "fundamentally wrong." In April 2017, he called legalization "a battle about sovereignty over our minds and bodies."

I interviewed Nadelmann repeatedly for this book. I liked him. He's not trying to get rich off legalization. And his concerns are impossible to discount. Maybe the racial disparities in marijuana arrests are so overwhelming that every other factor pales. Maybe we should let people find pleasure where they can by using a drug that is only moderately dangerous to most adults, as we do with alcohol. After all, schizophrenia usually develops before 30. No one disputes that occasional use of marijuana by people over 25 is generally safe.

But if Nadelmann and the rest of the marijuana lobby are so certain legalization is not just the right public policy decision but a moral imperative, why won't they be *honest* about the risks? Why won't they admit that legalizing marijuana, especially in its current high-THC form, amounts to running a giant real-time experiment on the brains of adolescents and young adults?

The reason, of course, is that they are trying to legalize a drug the United States has banned for eighty years. The Marijuana Policy Project brags, *"We change laws!"* And they know nothing would slow the rush to legalization faster than admitting that cannabis is connected to mental illness and violence, often of a particularly disturbing variety.

So, they offer the same circular argument as Taser did.

1. Marijuana doesn't cause schizophrenia.
2. It never has.
3. It never will.
4. Therefore, marijuana can't have caused this person to become psychotic, or the violence that followed.
5. Therefore marijuana doesn't cause schizophrenia.

But it does.

Researchers are still trying to figure the magnitude of the risks. They agree the connection between marijuana and psychosis is not as strong as that between tobacco and lung cancer. The best guess is that adolescent marijuana use raises the risk of schizophrenia between two- and six-fold. The great majority of teenagers who use marijuana will not develop the disorder.

Still, the recent hospital data, the spike in serious mental illness among young adults in the 2017 federal survey, and the studies from Denmark and Finland are not comforting. Clinically meaningful psychosis — including schizophrenia, psychotic depression, and bipolar disorder with psychosis — probably affects as many as 4 percent of people, or 1 in 25. (That figure does not mean 4 percent of the population is psychotic at any time. Even people with severe schizophrenia are not ill all the time, thankfully. And some people with less severe forms of psychosis can control their symptoms with medication or even recover fully.)

Jim van Os, a Dutch psychiatrist and epidemiologist and the author of a 2002 study on cannabis and psychosis, suggests that in countries with heavy use, marijuana could already be responsible for as much as 10 percent of psychosis in all its forms. In other words, as many as one extra person in 250 may develop psychosis from cannabis use. Considering the 11 percent figure from the hospital data, van Os's estimate seems conservative, if anything.

Even at 10 percent, the numbers are striking. The United States is a big country. About 40 million Americans were born in the last decade. An increase of 0.4 percent in psychosis would mean an extra 160,000 of those kids will suffer debilitating mental illness by 2040 or so. Many thousands of those will wind up committing murder and other violent crime. That figure doesn't account for other mental health problems marijuana might cause, like depression or suicidality, or decreases in IQ or memory.

And though schizophrenia generally develops in the late teens or twenties, evidence is mounting that prolonged, heavy cannabis use can lead to psychotic disorders for previously healthy adults outside the normal window for the disease. Van Os's 2002 survey of Dutch adults showed that adult users were far more likely to develop psychosis than nonusers. A more recent study of newly diagnosed psychosis in states with high cannabis use showed a surprising number of adults over 30 receiving diagnoses. Given the soaring number of heavy users smoking high-THC cannabis or THC extracts, millions of adults may be putting themselves at risk.

No wonder the cannabis lobby has done everything it can to shout down discussion of this issue.

When I told friends I was writing this book, they sometimes asked if it was "balanced."

The short answer is no. Not balanced doesn't mean inaccurate, dishonest, or in any way untruthful. But if you want to read about the way marijuana legalization will provide jobs, or anecdotes from people who believe that smoking cured their celiac disease, or discussions of the relative merits of indica and sativa strains, this book will disappoint you.

Maybe I'm too cynical, but I believe most people smoke marijuana for the same reason they drink alcohol or use any other drug: because they like to get high. Because *we* like to get high. The impulse for intoxication and chemical euphoria lies at the core of what it is to be human. And getting high is fun — at least for a while. The difference between cannabis and every other drug is that an entire industry now trumpets marijuana's benefits, promising a high with no low, a reward without risks.

As a psychiatrist in Denver said to me, "Marijuana has a great brand."

I didn't see much need to discuss the reasons people might want to use cannabis. You already know what those are.

Using cannabis or any drug is ultimately a personal choice. What to do about legalization is a political decision. But whether marijuana is dangerous to the brain and can ultimately cause violence is a scientific question, with a hard *yes* or *no* answer.

We have that answer. It's time you heard it.

This book begins in Indian psychiatric

hospitals in the nineteenth century and covers 150 years of history and science: the first glimpses of the marijuana-psychosis connection, prohibition, and the way the legalization lobby turned the debate, the modern research that locked down the link between marijuana and schizophrenia, and finally the newest research on marijuana and violence.

Throughout, I play with my cards up. This book is a work of nonfiction, and except in one instance where it is expressly noted, I haven't changed any names or any facts about any cases. Every study I mention is publicly available, and the NYU professor has made the code he used for his data analysis available, too. I have tried to present the counterarguments and the views of advocates like Nadelmann as fairly as I can. I am well aware of the skepticism I face, and this issue is too important to offer anything but the most honest possible picture.

The science can be complicated, and the descriptions of violence awful to read. But this book is also the story of dedicated physicians and researchers, like Sir Robin MacGregor Murray and Dr. Marta Di Forti — a husband-and-wife team who live in London and are two of the world's leading experts on cannabis and psychosis. I first met them at a 2017 conference in Waterville, New Hampshire, about the effects of cannabis on the brain. Murray, a Scottish-born psychiatrist, has treated people with schizophrenia for forty years and seen the effects of ever-stronger marijuana firsthand. "For the first couple of decades of my life as a clinician, we never bothered about cannabis," Murray told me in Waterville. If family members asked, he would tell them, "No, it's an entirely safe drug."

As he saw more cases, Murray began to wonder if the connection was coincidence. Now he is sure it isn't. He has tried to warn the world — with success in Britain, though not the United States. Psychiatrists like Murray (and my wife) are the main dissenting voices on this issue. They see the pain of psychosis up close. And they see firsthand how cannabis worsens the disease.

But Murray is an exception. Scientists and physicians rarely take center stage in public policy debates. They speak in the cautious language of scientific inquiry. And they're busy treating patients. Meanwhile, the marijuana lobby shouts: legalize, and everyone wins — except pharmaceutical companies and prison guards. No wonder the people who know the truth have so much trouble being heard.

I hope this book will be their bullhorn.

■ ■ ■ ■

PART ONE:
THEN AND NOW

■ ■ ■ ■

ONE:
MADNESS ON TWO CONTINENTS

A century ago, India and Mexico didn't have much in common.

India was the world's second most populous country, with 330 million people in 1900. It was mostly Hindu, was a British colony, and had a long history of cannabis use. Taxes and fees on the plant, which the British called Indian hemp, were a major source of government revenue.

Meanwhile, Mexico had a mere 13 million people. It was Catholic, independent, and new to cannabis. The plant was not native to the Western Hemisphere. Spanish colonizers had brought it, though they were largely unaware of its potential as a drug. They used its fibers for rope and ship rigging. Cannabis wasn't a major industry. Many Mexicans thought of it as a drug used mainly by soldiers and the poor.

Nine thousand miles separated the two countries. They had few connections.

Yet as the end of the nineteenth century approached, both struggled with the same question: Could the drug that Indians knew as *bhang, ganja,* or *charas,* and Mexicans called marihuana or Rosa Maria cause mental illness and violence?

The people of both India and Mexico were certain the answer was yes.

In 2012, Isaac Campos, a University of Cincinnati professor, wrote a book on the history of Mexican attitudes toward cannabis. The marijuana lobby in the United States portrays the drug war in Mexico as an outgrowth of American drug laws. Legalizers say the United States has exported its prohibitionist attitudes south.

The theory sounds good. It's become the conventional wisdom. There's only one problem. It's not true.

If anything, the opposite is the case. In his meticulously reported history, *Home Grown: Marijuana and the Origins of Mexico's War on Drugs,* Campos found that in the late 1800s — a period when few Americans had heard of marijuana — people in Mexico believed it caused mental illness and crime. Mexican newspapers portrayed marijuana users as prone to violence and self-injury.

In 1901, for example, a newspaper reported on a man who attacked strangers on a street and then "turned on himself and with bites he tore apart his own arms until a straitjacket could be put on him . . . he was crazy under the influence of marihuana."

Campos found hundreds of articles offering similar tales. Mexican doctors of the time who researched the drug agreed with the premise. None "rejected the basic view that it caused madness and violence."

Poor Mexicans were more likely to smoke marijuana than the wealthy. But fear of the drug did not stem from class prejudice. Poorer Mexicans were also concerned about marijuana's effects. The negative attitude toward cannabis was striking because people in Mexico had experience with psychotropic plants, including peyote and salvia, a type of sage that can produce hallucinations. They had no cultural reason to view marijuana negatively.

Yet they did. As marijuana's use spread, Mexicans viewed it as different from other drugs. It didn't merely cause users to hallucinate, like other psychotropics. Or excite them, like cocaine. Or disinhibit them, like alcohol. Instead, especially in large doses, it produced all three effects at once. It led to a delirium indistinguishable from insanity and often accompanied by violence. Newspapers regularly referred to criminals "as either a madman or a marihuano," Campos wrote.

Year by year, opposition increased. Mexican criminal defendants regularly claimed marijuana had driven them temporarily insane and that they shouldn't be held responsible for their actions. In one notorious case, the governor of Mexico City claimed in 1913 he had been high when he murdered a political rival.

Finally, in January 1920, the Mexican government found that marijuana was "one of the most pernicious manias of our people" and "not a medicine." On March 2, 1920, Mexico banned the sale of marijuana, along with cocaine and opiates. The latter two drugs were already becoming the subject of international narcotics control policies. But cannabis was still largely under the radar in Europe and the United States, Campos noted in his book. "Marijuana's inclusion was clearly Mexico's own contribution."

On the other side of the globe, Indians and their British overlords also worried about the effects of the pungent weed.

Indians prepared cannabis in three ways. They ground the plant's leaves and stems into a low-THC paste called bhang, which they then mixed into milk shakes — *bhang lassi* — which they drank at Hindu religious festivals.

Bhang was the most common drug made from cannabis. But Indians also smoked the plant's flowers, which they called ganja. Enterprising farmers in India had discovered the key to growing potent cannabis was to destroy the male plants in a batch. The remaining plants, all females, would try to attract males by growing larger flowers coated with a sticky resin high in THC. Farmers and smokers knew the resin was the most psychoactive part of the plant. (Across the globe, Mexican cultivators had reached the same conclusion. They called their high-potency marijuana *sinsemilla,* Spanish for "without seeds.")

Even more potent than ganja was a paste called *charas,* the Indian equivalent of hashish. Farmers made charas by rubbing resin from the flowers. Charas was usually smoked, though it could also be eaten.

British colonial records offer fascinating detail about the way Indian hemp was farmed and traded. The plants required careful handling to grow their resin-coated flowers. In Bengal, the biggest province, seedlings were planted in September. In

October laborers weeded the fields and in November pruned the seedlings to encourage their growth. Then a "ganja-doctor" arrived to separate the plants by sex. Harvesting and pressing the flowers to produce smokable ganja took place in February and March.

Cannabis cultivation was the lifeblood of the economy in some rural areas. It gave poor farmers the chance to raise a cash crop for sale, while provincial governments took their cut with taxes and licenses.

British colonizers took little notice of India's cannabis habit at first. In this neglect, they mirrored attitudes at home. In the nineteenth century, cannabis was hardly used in the United Kingdom. The British were far more interested in opium and its derivatives, like laudanum. Those drugs were popular, despite concerns about their potential for addiction and overdose.

But that hands-off attitude began to change by the 1860s. The British had brought what they called lunatic asylums to Indian cities.

And before long the British army doctors running them noticed that many patients had something in common. They or their families blamed their insanity on cannabis.

The trend became clear to colonial officials, too. Like all good colonizers, the British loved bureaucracy and record-keeping. Asylums published patient rosters that included the causes of admission, and "ganja" was commonly listed. In 1873, the government's financial department wondered if it should restrict cannabis use. It asked provincial officers if they had seen a connection between cannabis, insanity, and violence.

On December 17, 1873, the department published the survey results, providing what is probably the first official link anywhere between cannabis and mental illness. The report found "habitual use does tend to produce insanity." Still, the British officials called prohibition impractical. Instead, they recommended higher taxes "to discourage the consumption of bhang and ganja."

But the issue refused to go away.

The hospital rosters piled up. So did reports of brutal crimes. By 1891, a British politician asked for an investigation of whether cannabis might be more dangerous than opium. On July 25, 1893, in response to the criticism, the British government convened a seven-member group to examine cannabis in India. The Indian Hemp Drugs Commission included four British officials and three Indians, a breakdown that ensured that the colonizers would control its findings.

The commission heard testimony from 1,193 witnesses. It checked asylum reports and cultivation methods. It even asked a doctor to examine the effects of ganja on a rhesus monkey — who at first resisted being forced to enter a smoke-filled chamber but quickly became "restless and uneasy" on days when he wasn't allowed inside, and twice escaped his cage and tried to enter the chamber on his own.

On August 6, 1894, the commission issued its report, a massive document — 361 pages plus six volumes of appendixes. It found that the link between cannabis, insanity, and violence had been overstated. Some cases that asylum records reported as cannabis-related stemmed from opium and alcohol.

The report found that India should not prohibit bhang, ganja, and charas. Instead, the government should tax and regulate the drugs. One hundred twenty years later, marijuana advocates still cheer the commission's findings. Cannabis Digest, a Canadian site, wrote in 2014 that:

Marijuana historians and activists rightly regard this commission as a high point in cannabis scholarship. Published in seven volumes, and featuring interviews with a wide range of Indians plus others, it spoke with the voice of reason. It concluded that when used in moderation, ganja, as the locals called it, was benign.

Not exactly.

The British commissioners were happy to keep cannabis — and its tax revenue — legal. But two of the three Indian members disagreed. The sharpest dissent came from Lala Nihal Chand, a Punjabi lawyer. In a 120-page critique published on September 13, 1894, Chand took apart the commission's report. The commission had failed to distinguish between bhang, the low-THC product made from cannabis leaves, and high-THC ganja and charas, he said.

Of course, Chand never referred to THC, marijuana's main psychoactive ingredient. Chemists would not discover THC's exact structure until 1964. They would not find the brain receptors it affected until even later.

But everyone agreed that bhang was far less potent than the other preparations. The testimony before the commission also proved that Indians used bhang differently too, Chand wrote. Ordinary Indians drank *bhang lassi* during occasional religious festivals, enjoying the mild intoxication the milk shakes produced.

On the other hand, ganja and charas smokers were often daily users. Other Indians viewed them with disdain. Chand counted 638 witnesses who had testified against the two drugs. Only 26 had favored them. He even placed in the record folk sayings about the drugs: He who smokes ganja forgets even his own father's name. He is a charas smoker; you can't depend on him.

Chand then turned to the question of whether the drugs could cause mental illness. The committee's majority report had emphasized the fact that when it reexamined 222 cannabis-related asylum admissions in 1892, it had found that the real number was only 98. Asylum officers felt pressed to come up with a cause for admission and misclassified cases, the majority said.

But Chand pointed out that almost half of all admissions in 1892 the asylum reports listed the cause of insanity as "unknown." That fact alone suggested officials hardly felt pressure to insist on a cause when they couldn't find one.

In reality, statistics consistently showed that 20 to 30 percent of asylum patients were ill because of cannabis, he wrote.

Chand also noted that about 20 percent of the "criminal lunatics" in the Bengal asylums had a diagnosis of cannabis-related insanity, far more than those whose mental illness was attributed to alcohol or opium. He quoted doctors, police officers, and judges — both Indian and British — who linked the drug to violent crime.

"I know of a case in which an excessive ganja-smoker killed a friend of his with a lathi (a bamboo stick) without any apparent cause," one said. Another reported on a man "who consumed charas in considerable quantities, took a boy and deliberately chopped off his head. When kept out of the way of any hemp drugs, this man seems to behave fairly like a rational being; but whenever he gets charas, he gets violent and dangerous."

Chand disagreed with the commission's British majority. Low-potency bhang should remain legal, he wrote. But he called for ganja and charas to be prohibited, following a transition period to allow users the chance to quit the drugs.

A second Indian commissioner, Raja Soshi Sikhareswar Roy, agreed. "The prohibition of the use of ganja and charas would be a source of benefit," he wrote. But Chand and Roy couldn't overrule their colonial counterparts. All three forms of cannabis remained legal.

Even then the debate in India didn't end. British physicians kept seeing cases of mental illness and violence linked to the drug — and they refused to stay silent.

In 1904, Dr. George Francis William Ewens, the superintendent of the Punjab Lunatic Asylum, made an extraordinary thirteen-page report to *The Indian Medical Gazette.* Titled "Insanity Following the Use of Indian Hemp," the paper began:

There is a special form of mental disease met with in India usually classed as Toxic Insanity which seems to have a direct relation to the excessive use of hemp drugs . . . The symptoms are almost entirely mental, among the large number I have now seen, unlike the results of alcohol, arsenic, etc.

Ewens was both a stiff-upper-lip British military officer and a dedicated physician-scientist. Born in 1864, he received his MD from the Royal University of Ireland in 1888. Three years later, he graduated from the British Army Medical School and was appointed a surgeon in Bengal.

He spent the rest of his life in the army's

Indian Medical Service, becoming a lieutenant-colonel in 1911. He died on September 9, 1914, in Lahore, a dusty city in the northwest corner of British India (now part of Pakistan). He's buried there, under a long white gravestone. "Erected by his brother officers of the Indian Medical Service in token of their affection and esteem," his memorial reads.

Ewens seems to have devoted his life to his work; there's no record of his ever marrying or having children. In 1900, he became the superintendent of the asylum in Lahore. He ran it for a decade, getting a close look at insanity in all its forms. The emerging science of mental illness fascinated him. So did the relationship between mental illness and crime.

In 1908, Ewens wrote a 400-page book — in the preface, he charmingly called it "this little work" — called *Insanity in India: Its Symptoms and Diagnosis, with Reference to the Relation of Crime and Insanity.* He dedicated the book to a professor at King's College London — which coincidentally is now home to some of the world's top research on cannabis and mental illness.

But even before his "little work" in 1908, Ewens contributed to *The Indian Medical Gazette.* The *Gazette* was an English-language journal where officers and physicians reported on everything from "An Extraordinary Series of Outbreaks of Plague" to "Operating Rooms in the Tropics." (Until a few years ago, the *Gazette* would have been effectively lost to history, available only in a few university libraries. Today its issues are online in searchable PDFs.)

In the *Gazette*'s November 1904 issue, Ewens wrote to detail the relationship he had seen between cannabis and mental illness. Ewens knew the Indian Hemp Drugs Commission had criticized hospitals like his for blaming cannabis for insanity. His response was exceedingly British.

He lauded the commissioners for their "sincere conclusions," then added that "the smallest practical experience of insanity" proved them wrong. His hospital officers double-checked cases after admission. "There can be little mistake as to the fact of the habit; one often verified by the statements of friends and relations and confessed to by the man himself."

Patients whose insanity was due to cannabis also looked and acted different than others, Ewens wrote. "The cases of insanity attributed to hemp drugs excess show always a wonderful and most striking uniformity of symptoms." Those included hallucinations, delusions, and incoherent speech, which Ewens classified as "mania" and modern psychiatrists would call psychosis. He regularly saw cases of patients who recovered, were discharged, used again, and were readmitted. "Others who have strictly abstained have remained sane."

Ewens reported that at his hospital, 161 of 543 male patients — or 30 percent — owed their illness to cannabis. If the drug could cause mental illness, why did anyone use it? "The immediate effects of any very large dose of hemp is, first, dizziness followed by excitement, delirium, hallucination of a pleasant [sic] nature, a rapid flow of ideas, a state of ecstasy," Ewens wrote. Many Indians also viewed the drug as an aphrodisiac. But it also produced delusions, grandiose thoughts, and "a marked tendency to acts of willful damage and violence."

Good news, bad news, then.

As for treatment, "the absolute stoppage of all hemp drugs" offered the only cure, Ewens wrote. "I have never yet found any drug of the slightest service." Leeches and "blisters to the neck" were also useless.

Unfortunately, quitting was difficult. Unlike alcohol or opium, abstaining from cannabis did not produce physical withdrawal symptoms. "No ill-effects follow its sudden forcible stoppage," Ewens wrote. But despite the lack of physical symptoms, regular users craved the drug and gave it up with great difficulty.

Ewens finished by offering capsule reports on 95 patients, many of whom had committed violence and all of whom had symptoms that would be sadly familiar in any psychiatric hospital today:

No. 4 . . . Killed a man without provocation or apparent object, incoherent speech, fits of excitability, delusions of devatas (gods) to eat with him and that a man long dead comes each night . . .

No. 20 . . . Addicted to large quantities of bhang which he is even now asking for. Delusions of being an important paid servant of the asylum, very quarrelsome . . .

No. 41 . . . One day after an excess of charas threw his sister's child from the roof of a house killing her. Mania remained, sane for some years, and then after, it is believed having obtained some charas, quite suddenly, within a few hours, became acutely maniacal . . . Now again sane. No members of family ever insane . . .

Ewens wasn't the last British physician in India to link marijuana and mental illness. In 1914, Captain A. S. M. Peebles, another superintendent, published his own study in the *Gazette,* examining admissions at the Berhampore Lunatic Asylum.

Of 1,163 cases, 312 — or about 27 percent — were related to cannabis use, almost evenly divided between "criminal" and "non-criminal lunatics." In 24 cases, the patients had committed murder.

Like Ewens, Peebles took pains to argue that the statistics were accurate. They were based not just on admission reports, but on symptoms and statements the patients themselves had made, he wrote.

But most mentally ill ganja smokers remained in the community, Peebles wrote. "They are only ultimately sent to asylums when they have offended against the law or else become such intolerable nuisances." Thus, hospital admission statistics gave only a partial picture "of the extensive harm caused by the use and abuse of the drug."

The reports might be easy to dismiss as the biased work of British doctors hoping to ban cannabis. But the doctors took no position on that issue. They were simply reporting what they saw.

And what they saw remained strikingly

constant for fifty years. At least one in five patients in Indian mental hospitals had cannabis-linked illness. Neither alcohol nor any other drug was blamed nearly as frequently.

Many of those patients were ill only temporarily; they had what psychiatrists would now call "cannabis-induced psychosis." They recovered quickly and were sent home. Others were more seriously ill, with what would likely now be diagnosed as schizophrenia or bipolar mania. They remained hospitalized for months or years.

The statistics for what the doctors called "criminal lunatics" remained similar, too, with 20 percent or more of violence linked to cannabis use. The capsule case histories are depressingly familiar today, recounting unprovoked violence against family members and strangers.

Nor can the findings be dismissed as the product of Western doctors misunderstanding the cannabis-using customs of a foreign culture. Indian patients brought to asylums were not witch doctors acting out rituals that the British didn't understand. Family members often demanded their admission, the case reports show.

In the late nineteenth and early twentieth centuries, many Americans and Europeans had not even heard of cannabis. Few had used the drug. India had far more cannabis users than any other country. Whatever their flaws, the asylum rosters provide a unique resource, the first hard evidence of the relationship between the drug and mental illness.

Much more would come.

TWO:
SCHIZOPHRENIA, (MIS)UNDERSTOOD

George Francis William Ewens wasn't the only physician trying to understand mental illness in the late nineteenth and early twentieth centuries. Doctors were just beginning to categorize the brain disorders that caused people to disconnect from reality.

For millennia, people who talked to spirits, or heard voices, or acted strangely because of thoughts they couldn't control were called witches or demons. They faced cruel punishments and even crueler "treatments." The first step toward modern understanding came in 1841, when a German doctor named Karl Canstatt coined the term *psychosis* — short for *psychic neurosis,* or brain disease. Canstatt was trying to connect problems in the brain with crises of the mind, to understand how misfiring neurons might lead to failures of thought.

In "Insanity in India," Ewens offered as good a definition of mental illness as any:

Insanity is a disease of the brain causing an alteration or impediment of the mind, and by so doing altering a person's conduct, speech, manner and habits from those of sane people or of himself prior to his illness.

But what caused the changes? Doctors couldn't be sure:

Up to the present careful examination of the brains of most insanes after death has discovered nothing certain to which insanity can be attributed.

Still, Ewens was confident scientists would solve the puzzle:

Undoubtedly this is due to our defective powers of observation, and in all probability, it is only a question of time before such will be discovered.

More than a century later, Ewens's optimism has proven unfounded. Understanding what is going wrong in a person suffering from psychosis is complicated enough. Fixing it is even harder. After all, consciousness itself exists within the brain; I think therefore I am. We laugh and run and fall in love thanks to the interplay of electrical impulses in our heads. They form our perception of external reality. People having psychotic hallucinations don't lose their senses. But their brains overlay another layer of sight and sound atop the external stimuli the rest of us share. Those with delusions don't stop thinking, but they can't cross-check their thoughts against reality.

Rewiring the brain to undo those failures is far beyond us even now. Modern drug treatments for psychosis and schizophrenia are only moderately useful. Now called anti-psychotics, they were originally known as major tranquilizers because they are more knockout drugs than anything else. They blunt hallucinations and delusions but rarely eliminate them. They do even less to help schizophrenia's so-called negative symptoms, such as apathy and depression, or its cognitive symptoms. Besides everything else, schizophrenia damages memory and intelligence, and the losses grow with time. John Nash, the schizophrenic mathematician made famous in *A Beautiful Mind,* is very much the exception.

But when Ewens was practicing medicine, effective treatment wasn't even a dream.

Doctors were still working to classify mental illness. In 1893, a German psychiatrist named Emil Kraepelin coined the term *dementia praecox* — premature dementia — to explain why his patients suffered strange thoughts and visions in their teens and twenties.

A continent away from Kraepelin, Ewens was aware of the new term. In *Insanity in India,* he wrote, "There is a well-marked form of mental disease with special features termed by some Dementia Praecox." He defined its symptoms:

A gradual change of disposition; a loss of activity and energy, the patient becoming silly, shy, irritable, obstinate and careless; unable to follow his occupation or, if it begins more rapidly, doing so usually with a period of depression, apprehension, and suspicion, with it may be a foolish attempt at suicide. The combination of this condition with some silly senseless delusion and hallucination, especially of hearing (more rarely of sight), being typical of the disease.

A modern psychiatrist would recognize a patient with those symptoms as having schizophrenia. Ewens didn't use the term, because it hadn't been invented yet. It first entered the medical lexicon on April 24, 1908, when a psychiatrist named Eugen Bleuler used it in a talk to the German Psychiatric Association. It meant "split mind," and doctors rapidly adopted it for patients who had broken from reality.

Perhaps the most important characteristic of schizophrenia was the youth of its sufferers. As their peers were becoming adults, they lost their way. But even as children, before their symptoms bloomed into outright psychosis, they often seemed different. They might be socially maladjusted, intellectually impaired, or prone to violence. Sometimes they were all three.

Another defining characteristic was that treating schizophrenia was next to impossible. Early psychiatrists tried hypnosis, opiates and other drugs, and talk therapy. Nothing worked. Crueler treatments such as lobotomies or electroconvulsive therapy sometimes controlled symptoms for a while. But they rarely fixed the underlying disease.

Nonetheless, psychiatrists kept trying, because the pain psychotic disorders caused was so obvious, and because patients rarely improved on their own.

The schizophrenia diagnosis was useful, but it also proved problematic. It covered many symptoms. Some patients mainly had cognitive problems. They appeared more like people suffering from severe intellectual disability. Others had higher IQs but poor impulse control and a tendency to violence. They looked more like psychopaths. Still others fit the classic mode, with paranoia, delusions, and hallucinations.

Still, for lack of a better alternative, schizophrenia became the umbrella diagnosis psychiatrists gave people suffering from mental illness with psychotic features. Depression and manic depression — later called "bipolar disorder" — became the catchall diagnoses for people whose mental illness was centered around their mood. (Those lucky folks who were psychotic and depressed were called schizoaffective.)

Even though schizophrenia and psychosis went together, people could have psychotic episodes for many reasons, including tumors, strokes, and Parkinson's disease. As Ewens noted, one reason that doctors were so convinced that diseases of the mind occurred because of problems in the brain was that "insanity follows sometimes on brain injury."

Beyond physical trauma to the brain, extreme stress — such as being victimized by severe violence — could cause people to break from reality. So could manic episodes in which people went days without sleep, or even severe and long-term depression.

Drugs and chemicals, whether used recreationally or for medicinal purposes, could also make the brain go haywire. "All nations have some drug whose habitual use leads to dangerous consequences," Ewens wrote in *Insanity in India.* He judged cocaine more dangerous to the brain than opium and noted that alcohol too could cause psychosis.

So, a single psychotic episode didn't necessarily mean someone was schizophrenic. Over time, psychiatrists refined the diagnosis, recognizing its potential to stigmatize patients. Before calling a patient schizophrenic, psychiatrists had to rule out other potential causes. And the label should not be given quickly. A patient needed to have delusions or hallucinations that lasted months. Patients with less severe symptoms were called schizophreniform or schizotypal.

In other words, even experienced psychiatrists could argue over the diagnosis. One doctor might focus on psychotic symptoms and call a patient schizophrenic. Another might think the psychosis was secondary to a manic episode and say he was bipolar. Even now no blood tests or brain scans tell apart the diseases.

But by whatever name, people suffering from repeated psychotic episodes clearly needed treatment. From 1900 to 1950, that treatment came in the form of removal from the community and institutionalization. People with schizophrenia, severe depression, or bipolar disorder were permanently committed to state-run hospitals. To house them, Western nations went on a hospital-building spree. By 1955, the United States kept more than 550,000 patients in psychiatric hospitals, including 300,000 diagnosed with schizophrenia.

Some facilities were well managed and provided decent care. Others were little more than warehouses where desperately sick people moldered until they died. A few were worse, degrading patients and staff alike. But without effective medicines, doctors saw no alternative to long-term confinement.

Then, in December 1950, a French army surgeon looking for chemicals to reduce the physical stress of surgery discovered a compound called chlorpromazine. The new drug proved effective as a tranquilizer. In tests, it reduced body temperature and blood pressure, prolonged sleep, and made patients less anxious.

In this way, chlorpromazine was similar to older sedatives called barbiturates. But unlike barbiturates, it didn't produce euphoria or dangerously slow patients' breathing, so it was less likely to be abused or cause lethal overdoses. Physicians immediately saw its potential. It was first sold in France in 1952 under the name Largactil.

By then, two French psychiatrists had already discovered that chlorpromazine calmed their psychotic patients in ways that other drugs did not. It did not simply sedate them as barbiturates did. It actually reduced the intrusiveness of their hallucinations. In May 1952, they began to present their findings. The realization that the drug might offer a truly novel treatment for psychosis spread quickly.

Chlorpromazine's influence in the United States was especially revolutionary. Influenced by Freud's theories, American psychiatrists had tried for decades to cure schizophrenia with talk therapy. They had failed. Elite academic psychiatrists wanted to know if a patient was hallucinating because "of unconscious conflict over incestuous urges or stealing from his brother's piggy bank at the age of five," *Time* magazine snarkily wrote in March 1955. The correct answer: who cared? Unlike endless analysis, chlorpromazine actually helped psychotic patients.

Smith Kline & French, which sold the drug in the United States under the name Thorazine, wasn't shy about saying so. One creepy ad featured an oversized eye and the line, "When the patient lashes out against 'them,' Thorazine quickly puts an end to his violent outburst." Doctors reached for their prescription pads. Thorazine had $75 million in sales in 1955, its first full year on the market. In a 2005 history of chlorpromazine published in the *Annals of Clinical Psychiatry*, a Spanish psychiatrist called it "one of the greatest advances in twentieth-century medicine."

Chlorpromazine's success led pharmaceutical companies to introduce competing medicines with similar chemical structures and effects. The new drugs broke the grip of psychosis on patients. Keeping them hospitalized suddenly seemed unfair, unnecessary, possibly unconstitutional — and expensive. At first only a few patients were released, but year by year the momentum for deinstitutionalization grew. Books such as *One Flew Over the Cuckoo's Nest* and investigative reports like Geraldo Rivera's 1972 exposé of the filthy conditions at the Willowbrook State School, an institution for disabled children in New York, contributed to the pressure.

By 1980, the number of psychiatric inpatients had shrunk in the United States to 132,000 — a 75 percent decline in just twenty-five years. Europe saw similar trends. Ultimately, Thorazine and its chemical cousins gave more than a million mentally ill people a chance to leave psychiatric hospitals.

Unfortunately, the drugs proved to be less than the perfect treatments they had seemed at first. They frequently caused ugly movement disorders. Patients involuntarily smacked their lips or jerked their arms and legs. The side effects worsened with time and could be irreversible. Patients also complained that the medicines did not so much end their psychoses as make them unable to care about their symptoms — or anything else. People taking Thorazine might no longer be delusional, but most still couldn't work or have meaningful relationships. Some wound up more depressed than they had been when they were hospitalized.

As a result, many patients refused to take the drugs consistently. Being "off your meds" became popular shorthand for suffering mental illness. Patients would suffer a psychotic episode, be hospitalized, and be medicated until their symptoms resolved. Then they would be sent home with a pill bottle. But eventually they would stop their medicines, have another psychotic episode, and be hospitalized again.

Even worse, the drugs seemed to produce a sort of resistance in many patients.

By the mid-1960s, scientists had found that the drugs primarily bound to receptors in the brain that were activated by dopamine. Dopamine is a naturally occurring chemical that connects the brain's nerve cells. Its release is related to desire and motivation, and it helps cause the feelings of pleasure that drugs, sex, and food produce.

Excessive dopamine release is also related to psychosis and schizophrenia, though scientists are still not entirely sure how. In the short term, Thorazine and other antipsychotics provided relief by blocking dopamine from attaching to neurotransmitter receptors. But some patients' brains responded to the blocked receptors by producing even more of them — thus increasing their sensitivity to dopamine.

Those unlucky patients seemed to build up a tolerance to the drugs and required higher doses. But the higher doses could worsen side effects. And if patients stopped taking their medicines, they suffered what became known as *rebound psychosis.* In other words, cycling on and off the drugs could leave people with schizophrenia in worse shape than they had been before. Yet the side effects encouraged cycling.

In the 1990s, pharmaceutical companies introduced several new antipsychotic medicines to great fanfare. These became known as the "atypical antipsychotics" and became among the best-selling drugs in the United States. But studies showed the new drugs were generally no more effective than the older ones.

But even after doctors realized that antipsychotic medicines were not cure-alls, the move toward deinstitutionalization didn't stop. Long-term institutionalization can cost $100,000 a year or more per patient. Few adults with schizophrenia have private insurance, so federal and state governments bear the cost. Managing patients in the community was far cheaper than leaving them institutionalized.

By 2015, the United States had fewer than 40,000 beds in psychiatric hospitals, a drop of more than 90 percent from sixty years before. Heavily supervised treatment in group homes made up some of the difference. Still, the drop represented a huge shift. Essentially, governments gambled that they didn't have to lock people with psychosis away to keep them from becoming nuisances — or dangers. When they were wrong? Family members, neighbors, and even strangers paid the price.

Alongside the frustrating search for treatments for psychosis came an equally halting search for their causes.

From the first, scientists knew severe mental illness had a genetic component. Long before James Watson and Francis Crick discovered DNA, it was obvious that madness ran in families. Over time, researchers quantified the risk. A person with a schizophrenic parent had about a 4 percent chance of the disorder, compared to the 1 percent figure usually used for the general population. One with a brother or sister with schizophrenia had a nearly 10 percent chance. Identical twins were at much higher risk; if one was schizophrenic the other had an almost 50 percent chance of being so — even if the two twins were raised apart. That finding led scientists to say that roughly half the risk of schizophrenia was genetic.

Further research showed that calling the risk genetic wasn't quite accurate. Identical twins didn't just share genes. They shared the same womb, and prenatal factors also played a role in the disease. Children born to mothers who'd been undernourished or suffered a viral illness during pregnancy were more likely to be schizophrenic. Amazingly, even the season of birth seemed to matter. Large epidemiological studies showed that children born in the winter had a slightly higher chance of developing the disease. The difference was small but consistent across countries.

So, the 40 percent to 50 percent inborn risk of schizophrenia encompassed both genes and the prenatal environment. It represented the risk predetermined not from conception, but birth, an important distinction for researchers — though one that didn't help people at risk. They couldn't change their prenatal environments any more than they could swap out their genes.

In the 1990s, as scientists decoded the human genome — the strands of DNA that hold the information that eventually becomes us — psychiatrists hoped that they might find the genetic basis for that risk. But the genomes of people with schizophrenia or bipolar disorder didn't contain a smoking gun. Some rare brain disorders, like Huntington's disease, could clearly be linked to a single genetic mutation. But common mental illnesses were more like cancers, complex diseases that developed due to both genetics and environment. Like cancers, they were "associated with" dozens of genetic variations, not caused by one or two.

As for the other 50 percent to 60 percent of the risk, the cases that genes and prenatal biology could not explain? Clearly, those stemmed from factors after birth, whether in infancy, childhood, or adolescence. Every psychiatrist had a theory. People with schizophrenia were notoriously heavy cigarette smokers. But studies ultimately showed smoking resulted from rather than caused the disease. People with schizophrenia smoked because nicotine improved their alertness and lessened the side effects from antipsychotic drugs. Besides, most people with schizophrenia didn't care much about smoking's health risks. They had bigger problems.

Other psychiatrists noted that vitamin deficiencies seemed common in people with schizophrenia. Again, though, the relationship seemed to run the other way. Most schizophrenics ate badly — and sometimes wouldn't eat at all if they believed their food might be poisoned.

Other theories were even more dubious. In the 1930s, '40s, and '50s, many psychiatrists blamed bad mothers for schizophrenia. (Yes, really.) Studies seemed to suggest that schizophrenic patients had mothers who were either "overprotective," rejected them, or both. In 1948, the psychiatrist Frieda Fromm-Reichmann coined the term "schizophrenogenic" mothers. Mothers who rejected their children bred distrust that blossomed into paranoia, she theorized.

The theory persisted into the 1960s, despite growing evidence of the biological underpinnings of schizophrenia. Only when larger studies found no evidence that the mothers of people with schizophrenia had any particular parenting style — good or bad — did the theory mercifully wither.

"The theory of the schizophrenogenic mother (now) seems hopelessly mistaken, and more than a little embarrassing," a 2013 article in the *AMA Journal of Ethics* proclaimed. But the article noted the theory still had negative effects. Its residue discouraged modern psychiatrists from discussing genuinely bad parenting decisions with the mothers and fathers of troubled children.

Researchers also looked at general environmental factors. Poverty and severe mental illness were highly connected. But epidemiologists found that poverty, like smoking, generally resulted from rather than caused mental illness. Most people with schizophrenia were unemployed and eventually slid into poverty even if they came from middle-class families.

Other studies consistently showed immigrants had higher rates of schizophrenia than native-born citizens. The immigration link remains tantalizing, but no one has fully explained it. In the United States, the fact that African Americans were more likely to be diagnosed with schizophrenia than white people led to fierce debate. Some researchers believed the gap reflected a true difference in disease rates. Others said that psychiatrists were simply more likely to label blacks, especially black men, as schizophrenic. White patients might be called bipolar with psychotic features — a diagnosis that carried less stigma. But even when psychiatrists used standardized checklists instead of relying on their own impressions to make diagnoses, the disparities remained.

A few researchers, usually psychologists or other nonphysicians, went further. They argued schizophrenia and psychosis were cultural constructs. Many patients didn't actually want or need help, they said. In 2014, a monograph from the British Psychological Society claimed, "There is no clear dividing line between 'psychosis' and other thoughts, feelings and beliefs" and argued that people who didn't want to think of themselves as being schizophrenic weren't, not really:

Some people find it useful to think of themselves as having an illness. Others prefer to think of their problems as, for example, an aspect of their personality which sometimes gets them into trouble but which they would not want to be without . . .
In some cultures, experiences such as hearing voices are highly valued.

Those pleasant-sounding theories bore little relationship to the painful realities that many people with psychosis face. The monograph also stated — flatly and incorrectly — that "It is a myth that people who have these experiences are likely to be violent." (Technically, they might not be likely to be violent, if *likely* is defined as "more than 50 percent," but they are far more likely than healthy people.)

Of course, some people with mild schizophreniform disorder were indistinguishable from people who simply had strange ideas about alien civilizations or political conspiracies. As long as they could function, their odd ideas hardly mattered. But people who came to the attention of emergency room doctors or police officers almost by definition were not functioning.

And doctors didn't need lectures on sensitivity to know they shouldn't find people mentally ill for acting in ways that were culturally or religiously reasonable. A Haitian who believed in voodoo was no more psychotic than a devout Catholic who believed in the intercession of the saints. As George Ewens wrote in the introduction to his book:

> Insanity in India is, of course, essentially the same as insanity anywhere else in the world, though its evidences equally, of course, are modified by the environment, habits and customs of the people.

Still, the fact that a society of British psychologists could argue in 2014 that schizophrenia might not even be real showed how little progress scientists had made since Emil Kraepelin invented the term *dementia praecox.* Despite a century of research, the disease's causes remained murky and its treatments marginally effective. But the pain it caused to sufferers and their families was as severe as ever.

As they considered bad mothering, cigarettes, and vitamin deficiency, researchers also wondered if recreational drugs might cause schizophrenia. They knew stimulants like cocaine regularly provoked psychotic episodes. Opiates could cause delirium, though full-on psychosis seemed less common.

Along with the British asylum reports, letters about cannabis popped up in other scientific journals too. In 1908, for example, the *Boston Medical and Surgical Journal* published a report from a physician at a mining camp in Mexico. "My little camp of 700 or 800 is a perfect clinic of hysteria . . . caused by smoking a weed, growing abundantly in the hills, called 'marihuana,' " he wrote. "[The] mania is extremely violent for two or three days, requiring enforced restraint: it is accompanied by hallucinations."

In general, though, physicians assumed that drug-induced psychoses were temporary. In fact, for most of the twentieth century, no rigorous studies showed that marijuana could cause permanent psychosis.

The weakness of the science is less surprising than it might seem. Before the 1970s, cannabis use was rare in Europe and the United States. A 1969 Gallup survey showed that only 4 percent of Americans said they had ever tried marijuana. Like cocaine and heroin, the drug hardly existed outside of big cities. It was used primarily by minority groups, and a handful of whites who self-identified as members of the counterculture — most famously jazz musicians.

Further, most American marijuana at the time was quite weak, containing only 0.5 percent to 2 percent THC. Mexican sinsemilla was expensive and uncommon, and hashish even rarer. Under those circumstances, THC's link to mental illness would had to have been incredibly strong for it to be visible on a population-wide basis.

So, the link between cannabis and mental illness remained scientifically unproven through the 1960s. Even so, lawmakers and their constituents agreed that cannabis, like cocaine and heroin, was a dangerous drug. In most states, selling even a few joints was a felony that could carry a long prison sentence — and dealing marijuana to a minor was theoretically punishable by death in some Southern states.

But that consensus was about to topple.

THREE:
GETTING HIGH IN THE 1970s

Even as fears about marijuana spread north from Mexico after 1910, the drug remained legal in the United States. Until 1937, the nation didn't even have a federal law restricting the drug. Plus, after 1920, police were focused on Prohibition, the doomed effort to make the United States a dry country.

But Americans quickly decided that banning the sale of alcohol was a mistake. Beer, wine, and whiskey had been part of American life for centuries. Prohibition made criminals of tens of millions of law-abiding adults. On December 5, 1933, it was officially repealed. Legal alcohol sales resumed. Police could focus their attention elsewhere.

Many Americans of the era had experience with opiates and cocaine. Those drugs had been widely used in over-the-counter "patent" medicines. Ordinary people knew they could be addictive and dangerous. They were less aware of marijuana's potential risks.

Harry J. Anslinger, the commissioner of the Federal Bureau of Narcotics, decided to inform them. Anslinger compiled reports on horrific crimes whose perpetrators had supposedly used marijuana and encouraged newspapers to write about them. The press eagerly took up the cause, despite the relative lack of scientific evidence at the time. (The irony deserves a mention. Today, far more evidence supports marijuana's link to mental illness and violence. Yet media outlets now take a cheery, credulous tone toward cannabis. That attitude is especially true in states where the drug is legal, and dispensaries and delivery companies can advertise. The *San Francisco Chronicle* even has an editor who both covers the industry and "develops new media products, services, and events in the cannabis space" — a conflict of interest that most newspapers would not have allowed when they were financially healthier.)

By 1937, Anslinger had won his fight. On August 2, President Franklin D. Roosevelt signed the federal Marihuana Tax Act into law. The law included a prohibitive $100-per-ounce tax on anyone who used cannabis for purposes other than very limited industrial or medical use. Combined with the spread of state laws against the drug, the tax act effectively made marijuana illegal in the United States.

For the next generation, most Americans didn't care much one way or the other, as Gallup's 4 percent survey figure showed. Because marijuana was so rarely used, arrests for the drug were confined to society's margins. Fewer than 19,000 Americans were arrested for marijuana possession or sale in 1965. No one else paid much attention to the penalties they faced.

But in the late 1960s, cannabis became central to a broader cultural conflict. With the war in Vietnam worsening and race riots tearing cities apart, many young Americans no longer trusted the government. They rejected not just the politics of the establishment but its cultural values. The two sides dressed differently, listened to different music, and even had their own drugs. For the establishment, those were alcohol and cigarettes. For the counterculture, marijuana and, to a lesser extent, hallucinogens like LSD. In his 1971 book *Marihuana Reconsidered,* Lester Grinspoon, a physician who became an advocate of legalization, neatly summarized the fight:

> Marijuana belongs to the younger genera-
> tion and is viewed by them and their elders
> as a symbol of youth's social alienation . . .
> Covert racism is probably another factor
> that inflames this issue . . . cannabis is
> viewed, perhaps largely unconsciously, as
> the nonwhite drug which is rapidly invad-
> ing the white community.

Grinspoon's arguments held more than a grain of truth. And the opposition to marijuana from President Nixon and other conservative politicians only encouraged young people to try it. As the counterculture spread, cannabis use surged.

By March 1973, 12 percent of Americans surveyed by Gallup said they had used the drug at least once — a tripling in three years. Among young people, use spread even faster. Half of all Americans aged 18 to 24 had used cannabis by 1975.

Perhaps even more importantly, a community sprung up to champion use of the drug, lash out at its critics, and lobby to end penalties against it. That development made marijuana unique among illegal drugs. Cocaine and heroin and methamphetamine had users; cannabis had proselytizers.

The passion of the drug's advocates became clear when Tom Forcade founded *High*

Times magazine in 1974. Forcade was one of the more fascinating characters the counterculture ever produced, an underground journalist who was also a big-time marijuana smuggler. Born Kenneth Gary Goodson in Phoenix, Arizona, in 1945, by the late 1960s he was calling himself Thomas King Forcade — his last name a play on *façade.*

Hugh Hefner and *Playboy* had helped liberalize the way Americans thought about sex. Forcade hoped *High Times* would do the same for cannabis and other drugs — though not heroin, which he said was "social control on a molecular level."

He was more successful than anyone could have imagined. "Forcade had seen a magazine audience that no one else knew existed: hard-core drug users," the journalist Patrick Anderson wrote in a 1981 book, *High in America.* "His magazine soon became slick and well-edited. Its model was *Playboy,* but its obsession was not sex, and its centerfolds featured ripe marijuana plants instead of ripe young women."

Soon *High Times* was selling almost a half million copies every month. The magazine took as a given the proposition that marijuana should be legal. It happily accepted advertisements for bongs and other smoking paraphernalia.

Unfortunately, Forcade suffered from mood swings and paranoia — no doubt both worsened by his drug use, as well as his second career as a smuggler. In a 1978 interview, he complained government agencies had "planted women informers to try to fuck me, they've planted informers in positions as *High Times* office boys, office managers, and accountants . . . Effectively, I've spent the last ten years in jail — I've been under such close surveillance."

Forcade killed himself with a gunshot to the head three weeks later at his downtown Manhattan apartment. After his cremation, his magazine's staff smoked his ashes on the top of the World Trade Center — the highest place they could find. But even without its founder, *High Times* pushed on, fighting for cannabis with every issue.

Working alongside *High Times* was the National Organization for the Reform of Marijuana Laws. A young Indiana lawyer named Keith Stroup had founded NORML in 1970. In a 1973 *New York Times Magazine* profile, Stroup explained he had created the group after seeing a friend arrested. "The only people working for reform then were freaks who wanted to turn on the world, an approach that was obviously doomed to failure. I wanted an effective, middle-class approach, not pro-grass but anti-jail."

For a time, Stroup wanted the *R* in NORML's name to stand for "Repeal," not "Reform." But surveys showed that fewer than 20 percent of Americans wanted marijuana to be legalized. Stroup settled on an incremental approach. Instead of legalization, NORML fought for decriminalization or at the least a softening of the laws on marijuana possession. Those could be draconian, especially in the South. The 1973 *Times Magazine* article explained that 691 people were imprisoned in Texas on marijuana possession charges, with an average sentence of more than nine years. It profiled some:

There was a very straight young man from a small town who was a cemetery-lot salesman and bowling instructor before being sentenced to five years on his second conviction for possessing a few ounces.

There was a husky Latin-American who had grown up in an orphanage and was about to enter college on a football scholarship when he was convicted for selling several ounces of marijuana; as he told the story, his judge, noting that he had no family, said, "Son, we'll give you a home," and then sentenced him to 40 years.

Such cases were becoming rarer. By 1973, simple marijuana possession was a felony in only two states, Texas and Rhode Island. Still, even a misdemeanor arrest could be punished by a year in jail. And the number of arrests had soared along with use of the drug. Between 1965 and 1973, arrests rose more than twenty-fold, to 420,000.

Suddenly, plenty of middle-class white people were getting picked up. For them, the laws against marijuana use were no longer merely a theoretical concern. Even folks who had never touched a joint could feel the sting if the police dragnet swept up their children. The arrests — and the incarceration that often followed — came as an unpleasant shock to people who figured they couldn't get in trouble for selling a few ounces to buddies. As the *Times Magazine* reported:

The [Texas] prisoners told depressingly similar stories: widespread marijuana use among their friends; an "It can't happen to me" attitude; arrest by undercover agents; lawyers who demanded huge fees and promised that there was nothing to worry about; headline-seeking district attorneys; and finally conviction; wives and children left behind; and the reality of long, long sentences.

Stroup and NORML found a ready audience for their message. In 1973, Oregon became the first state to decriminalize the possession of small amounts of marijuana. In 1975, four more states followed.

Support for marijuana and anger at those who enforced laws against it spread from the counterculture to become a staple of the center-left. In 1974, the *New York Times* ran a book review arguing that Drug Enforcement Administration agents "bully pot smokers with antiquated laws . . . sometimes enjoy framing innocent people; occasionally kill from what appears to be sheer whimsy or stupidity; waste millions of dollars annually; and regularly fail to perform their assigned task of stopping the hard-drug traffic."

By then, Watergate had made Nixon a national villain. When he resigned, marijuana advocates believed that the United States might move not just toward decriminalization, but full legalization.

The fact that marijuana didn't seem

particularly dangerous helped the cause. As advocates noted, Americans had been told that cannabis would drive them insane. Instead, many found the drug to be nothing more than a mild intoxicant. That personal experience led them to question everything they'd been told about marijuana.

There was only one problem: most of them were smoking the cannabis equivalent of near-beer. In the 1960s and 1970s, most marijuana used in the United States was cheap weed imported in bulk from Mexico, in some cases literally parachuted by the ton out of planes. The stuff was not just low in THC but often so jumbled with useless seeds and stems that users had to shake it out before they could smoke it.

Federal testing of seized marijuana at the time showed that it rarely contained more than 2 percent THC. Some legalization advocates now argue that testing techniques then underestimated the THC content, but Lester Grinspoon himself used "1 to 2 percent" as an estimate for the potency of American marijuana in his 1971 book. A 1972 federal study reported that "most marihuana available in this country comes from Mexico and has a THC content of less than 1%."

The math matters here. Bear with me.

An average joint weighs roughly a half gram. In other words, it contains about 500 milligrams of marijuana, an amount that hasn't changed much in half a century. But in a 1970s marijuana cigarette, THC — the active ingredient — accounted for only 1 percent to 2 percent of that weight.

Thus, an average joint then contained roughly 5 to 10 milligrams of THC. Burning the cigarette to produce the smoke destroys about half of that THC. So, the actual amount of THC available for inhalation in a typical 1970s joint was no more than 2.5 to 5 milligrams. Since new users generally shared joints rather than smoked alone, they were likely inhaling no more than 1 or 2 milligrams of THC per cigarette.

How small a dose is that? Cannabis advocates today generally suggest that 2.5 milligrams of THC is the equivalent of a single drink for a new or infrequent user. So even someone who has never used marijuana before will probably feel only slight psychoactive effects from a 1- to 2-milligram dose.

Because most 1970s marijuana was so weak, light smokers might as well have loaded their joints with oregano. At most, they would wind up slightly buzzed after sharing a couple of joints.

In his 1971 book, Grinspoon compared

American marijuana to bhang, the weakest Indian cannabis. The comparison was apt. Drinking a *bhang lassi* at a Hindu festival was as much a religious ritual as a serious effort at intoxication for many Indians. Similarly, taking a few hits of marijuana at a party or concert turned out to be a cultural statement as much as anything else for many Americans.

Of course, smoking enough weak marijuana to get high wasn't impossible, but it was work, in the same way that getting drunk on low-alcohol beer would be. On Internet message boards, older smokers recall going through an ounce of marijuana with four or five friends over the course of a night. At that rate, the group would share fifty joints so each smoker could reach a dose of 25 to 50 milligrams of THC. They'd be high. They'd also probably have sore throats from all the smoke and sore fingers from pulling the seeds.

(Today, marijuana is far stronger, regularly 20 percent to 25 percent THC. At that potency, a single joint can contain more than 100 milligrams of the drug. And regular smokers sometimes coat their joints with near-pure THC oil extracts, further increasing the amount of THC. The sharp rise in marijuana's THC content runs contrary to the arguments of legalizers that banning drugs encourages dealers to increase their potency because they can then smuggle less of the more concentrated substance. Demand from consumers, not growers or dealers, seems to have driven the move to higher-THC marijuana. Users prefer higher-THC forms of the drug because they can smoke less and get high more quickly. Smokers want to "party and get wasted," a grower told the online magazine *Slate* in a 2013 article about potency. The legalized market has responded to their wishes.)

For committed smokers of the 1970s, sinsemilla was available. But though it was significantly less potent than marijuana today, usually less than 10 percent THC, it was far more expensive. In 1977, sinsemilla could cost as much as $400 an ounce. Adjusted for inflation, that price is more than 15 times what an ounce of marijuana now costs in legal states. Most smokers were stuck with marijuana that barely contained THC at all.

The weakness of 1960s- and 1970s-era cannabis explains why so many articles of the time include stories of people saying they didn't feel anything when they smoked. Keith Stroup of NORML was one, at least at first. In his 1981 book about legalization, Patrick Anderson wrote that Stroup had "smoked marijuana a few times in law school without ever getting high."

Soon enough Stroup found more potent marijuana — and saw the drug's effects, and side effects, for himself. As Anderson wrote:

> He and Kelly [his wife] smoked while playing bridge with some friends . . . soon they were stoned, and the bridge game was forgotten. Keith rocked so obsessively in a rocking chair that the chair broke. Then he became convinced that someone was about to murder his and Kelly's new daughter, and he raced home to save her . . .
>
> Another time . . . Kelly prepared her specialty, roast duck, but they all got stoned before dinner, and someone dropped the duck, and then Stroup became paranoid, convinced that Ronnie (a friend of a friend who had come for dinner) was going to kill them.

In other words, even the director of NORML knew that when the drug was strong enough to get him high, it could easily make him paranoid, too.

Nixon's resignation paved the way for

Jimmy Carter to win the presidency in 1976. With a Democrat in the White House, marijuana seemed to be speeding toward national decriminalization. Stroup was close to Carter's top drug policy advisor, Dr. Peter Bourne. And four more states decriminalized in 1976 and 1977. In interviews, Stroup confidently predicted a dozen more might follow by 1980.

In a 1977 speech on drug abuse, Carter made the case for decriminalization: "Penalties against possession of a drug should not be more damaging to an individual than the use of the drug itself, and where they are, they should be changed."

Then Stroup and other advocates made a mistake. They let the world see how much they liked getting high. And they liked getting high a lot. Not only on cannabis, but on cocaine, an Ecstasy-like drug called MDA, and just about any other bit of chemical euphoria they could snort, swallow, or smoke.

Since the 1950s, scientists had debated the "gateway drug" hypothesis, the theory that smoking marijuana raised the risk for the later use of other drugs. In the one-man sample of Stroup himself, the answer was clear. He'd started with marijuana and ended with everything else. He wasn't alone, either. NORML staffers joked they would soon be changing the group's name to NORCL, with the *C* standing for cocaine.

In December 1977, Bourne, the White House drug advisor, used cocaine with Stroup and other people at NORML's annual party in Washington. (Bourne always denied using, saying he had only "held" a vial of cocaine before passing it on. His explanation never got much traction. As the old joke goes, *I don't do coke, I just like the smell.*) Seven months later, the story of Bourne's use leaked to the media. Stroup, who was angry at Bourne over a United States–backed program to spray herbicide on Mexican marijuana fields, didn't deny it. Bourne was forced to resign from the White House.

But for Stroup, Bourne's departure wasn't even a Pyrrhic victory. It was an instant defeat. The story linked cocaine and marijuana indelibly in the public mind at a time when cocaine use was exploding. A 1979 poll showed that 28 percent of adults 18 to 25 had used cocaine, triple the percentage in 1972.

Other surveys showed that marijuana use strongly predicted cocaine use. A high school senior in 1980 who had never used marijuana had only a 1-in-300 chance of using cocaine, according to research from the National Institute on Drug Abuse. If he'd smoked more than forty times, he had better than even odds. When it came to cocaine, at least, the gateway theory seemed plausible.

Reasonable people could debate the risks of cannabis. But no one except hard-core drug legalizers would defend cocaine. It produced euphoria followed by a quick crash. Users had to have strong self-control to avoid going back for more. Many people became rapidly addicted. It was so expensive that heavy users could bankrupt themselves in months. Cocaine was also physically dangerous, causing heart attacks and strokes.

The connection proved devastating for marijuana. Stroup had portrayed himself as a civil rights activist, fighting against long prison sentences. Now it seemed that he and other advocates simply wanted to encourage people to get high.

"I'm sure that if it hadn't been for the mass marketing of cocaine, marijuana would have been legalized," Glenn O'Brien, an editor at *High Times* during the 1970s, said in Martin Torgoff's 2004 book *Can't Find My Way Home: America in the Great Stoned Age, 1945–2000.*

Plus, by the late 1970s, a lot of parents had seen up close the way marijuana use affected their kids. They didn't like it. Even when it didn't lead to other drugs, cannabis seemed to hurt concentration, memory, and motivation.

Making matters worse, the booming drug paraphernalia industry regularly promoted its products to minors. Paraphernalia sales had exploded during the 1970s. "Head shops" sold rolling papers, bowls, brightly colored bongs, and traps where smokers could hide their stashes.

By 1978, the shops were established enough to have a lobbying group, the Paraphernalia Trade Association. In a December 1978 article, the *Washington Post* estimated the size of the market at $350 million annually — about $1.5 billion in today's dollars. The article was notable for its wink-and-a-nod attitude:

Step right up, folks! Take a look at the hottest thing on the market! It's an item every hip home should have, a unique "preparation system" to grind your favorite white, crystalline substance into a fine, snowy powder . . .

Right next to the pale green plastic device, which a reckless lawbreaker could possibly use for pulverizing cocaine, if such an idea should ever occur, we find a nifty kit to convert the knob on an automobile gear shift (floor model) to a pipe. Who knows what could be smoked in such a pipe, which comes complete with a long plastic tube for the driver's convenient inhalation. It is also only $14.95, and just in time for Christmas.

Many products, like a baby bottle that included both a nipple and a hash pipe, seemed designed to entice kids. On March 30, 1978, the *New York Times* reported that in a test, three boys and a girl aged 11 to 14 had bought paraphernalia at several shops. "No salesman turned down the four customers as being too young, they reported, even though they looked barely their ages," the *Times* wrote.

Store owners and employees seemed to regard the products as a joke. Parents didn't agree. To them, the paraphernalia encouraged their children to think of drugs as cute. Even parents who used themselves were shocked by the industry's attitude.

The combination of parental pushback and the Peter Bourne scandal effectively ended the decriminalization movement. By the end of 1978, Stroup had resigned as the head of NORML. The organization's lobbying effectiveness disappeared. The cultural, political, and legal pendulum swung against drug use. Over the next two decades, not one state would decriminalize.

Stroup and NORML had won when they framed their fight as about civil rights and fairness in law enforcement. Once they were perceived as advocates for getting high, the public turned on them.

The way to get traction for marijuana legalization was to make the argument about everything other than the reason that people used the drug. Stroup had realized that fact before anyone else. Then he'd forgotten — and his movement had paid the price.

Only in the 1990s would a new generation of legalizers arrive. They were far more careful, savvy, and better funded than Stroup had ever been. And they had learned from his mistakes.

FOUR:
THE FIRST REAL PROOF

As cannabis use surged in the late 1960s and '70s, psychiatrists who had rarely dealt with the drug before saw its effects up close — and reported their findings:

Forty-six cases of psychosis in cannabis abusers (*International Journal of the Addictions,* 1972).

Psychotic reactions following cannabis use in East Indians (*Archives of General Psychiatry,* 1974).

Cannabis-associated psychosis with hypomanic features (*Lancet,* 1982).

Cannabis psychosis in south Sweden (*Acta Psychiatrica Scandinavica,* 1982).

For the most part, the reports didn't make sweeping conclusions about marijuana's effects on the brain. Psychiatrists and emergency room physicians were simply trying to manage psychotic breaks in smokers. Did they need antipsychotic medicines? Or could they simply be left in seclusion until their hallucinations and delusions faded? Fortunately, the crises seemed temporary, at least in people without underlying mental illness. After a day or two, most patients calmed down.

At the same time, doctors saw cannabis provoking new psychotic episodes in people who already had schizophrenia. A 1978 case report in the *American Journal of Psychiatry* discussed four patients whose symptoms worsened when they smoked. "The sole substance abused was marijuana," the report said. "Each time marijuana use at moderate levels began, there was exacerbation and deterioration."

But many psychiatrists viewed the reports as a curiosity. Then as now, the specialty leaned to the left. In 1964, almost 1,200 psychiatrists had signed a letter arguing that Barry Goldwater, the Republican candidate for president, was "psychologically unfit" for the office. (The criticism that followed led the American Psychiatric Association to say none of its members should offer a diagnosis of a public figure unless he or she had examined the figure personally. Known as the "Goldwater rule," the restriction remains today.)

The dislike ran both ways. In his book *The Selling of the President,* the journalist Joe McGinniss recounted that Richard Nixon's campaign wouldn't let a psychiatrist on a panel that would question Nixon. "Nixon hates psychiatrists," a Nixon advisor told McGinniss.

Three years later, Nixon's own Oval Office tapes would catch him complaining to an aide about psychiatrists — specifically Jewish psychiatrists — and the nascent cannabis legalization movement:

> Every one of the bastards that are out for legalizing marijuana is Jewish. What the Christ is the matter with the Jews, Bob, what is the matter with them? I suppose it's because most of them are psychiatrists, you know, there's so many, all the greatest psychiatrists are Jewish . . .

Nixon was wrong, at least about the two men who would become the most important advocates during the 1970s. Neither Keith Stroup nor Tom Forcade was Jewish — or a psychiatrist. But the fact that psychiatrists like Lester Grinspoon were among the doctors best-known for favoring marijuana use couldn't be argued. (Grinspoon's cannabis advocacy makes him a hero to modern-day legalizers; there's even a marijuana strain called Dr. Grinspoon, "for connoisseurs and intellectuals." His similar work on behalf of cocaine has been forgotten; in 1978, he said cocaine was less dangerous than alcohol or tobacco and the penalties for its use much too harsh.)

The chasm between Nixon and psychiatry meant that many psychiatrists in the 1970s were in no hurry to sound an alarm on marijuana's potential dangers. But the debates about marijuana's risks in the 1970s suffered from an even more fundamental problem. Case reports don't prove anything. Yes, some people with schizophrenia broke down after smoking. But maybe others didn't. Without knowing the denominator, the numerator was meaningless.

Scientists make a distinction between "hypothesis-generating studies" and "hypothesis-testing studies." *Hypothesis* is a fancy word for theory. It's easy to generate a hypothesis: Maybe preservatives are good for you. They preserve hot dogs, don't they? Almost any theory can look plausible if you squint hard enough.

Figuring out whether the theory is true is

much harder, especially if the theory is that a drug or activity is harmful to the people who use it. Scientists can't ethically test something on people to see if it might hurt them. Ever since the disclosure of the repulsive experiments that German and Japanese scientists conducted during World War II, that restriction has been a core principle of medical research — and it should be.

The case reports on cannabis in the 1970s were hypothesis generating. By showing that cannabis could cause temporary psychosis, they raised the bigger question of whether the drug might have serious long-term effects, worsening or possibly even causing schizophrenia.

But for a decade, no one made any progress in testing that theory.

Then Sven Andréasson had an idea.

Andréasson is a Swedish physician who specializes in addiction medicine and alcoholism. He practices at the Karolinska Institute, the Stockholm medical university responsible for choosing the Nobel Prize in medicine each year.

In the early 1980s, Andréasson had just started practicing. He noticed that the schizophrenic patients who relapsed after being released from his hospital were often the ones who used cannabis. The patients came back "with much more florid hallucinations or disordered thinking," he told me. Of course, Andréasson wasn't the first doctor to wonder if cannabis might be connected to schizophrenia. But unlike everyone else, Andréasson and his supervisor, Peter Allebeck, had a way to test their theory.

At the time, Sweden had a military draft, with universal male conscription. Sweden being Sweden, this draft wasn't an American-style process that well-connected men could avoid. Practically every male Swede served. During the intake process, conscripts filled out two questionnaires, one about their education and upbringing, the other about drug use. The military used the information to figure out what jobs to give recruits. The questionnaires were saved, but the personally identifying information in them was supposed to be destroyed.

However, the questionnaires from the 1969–70 year hadn't had their identifiers removed. A Swedish military psychologist had wanted to create a database for future use, Andréasson said. But the psychologist never used the files. The tapes that contained their results sat moldering in a basement. They had been scheduled to be destroyed until Allebeck saved them.

When Allebeck mentioned the files, Andréasson realized their value. They covered almost fifty thousand conscripts, a full year's population of Swedish men. Under normal circumstances, a researcher would be thrilled to have a dataset one-tenth that size. Many studies cover only a few hundred people. But teasing out the factors behind an uncommon disease like schizophrenia is difficult without a big dataset — a random 2,000-person sample might include only 15 people who develop the disease.

Further, Andréasson didn't have to worry that the data might have a hidden bias because researchers hadn't attracted a fully representative sample. Every Swedish conscript had been surveyed, full stop. Ninety-two percent of those had filled out the survey about their drug use. The background questionnaire was comprehensive, too, as one would expect from a survey created for military use. And the men were the right age. They had mostly been born in 1951 and been 18 or 19 when they filled out the questionnaires. They'd come of age in the late 1960s, as marijuana use was rising, and been surveyed exactly when men began to develop schizophrenia.

"We had access to so much data about

these conscripts — there were hundreds of items in these questionnaires that they all answered," Andréasson said.

But the questionnaires were only half the puzzle. For them to mean anything, Andréasson had to have outcome data. In other words, he needed to know what had happened to the conscripts since they'd served, so that he could see which of them had wound up with mental illness. Fortunately, Sweden's national health care system gave him the chance to find out. Sweden tracks hospitalizations, and because the military surveys contained personal identifying data, Andréasson could see exactly which conscripts had been hospitalized.

"We had a complete inpatient registry for this group, and in particular a psychiatric inpatient registry, which in the case of schizophrenia is very good," Andréasson said. "If you really develop schizophrenia, you're likely to have been treated in a hospital." Even criminals wouldn't be missed, since Sweden screens prisoners for mental illness.

To be sure he had captured most cases, Andréasson sampled the inpatient registry. "We didn't take it for granted — we did a number of investigations." He found it was comprehensive.

He also checked the honesty of the self-reported drug use on the conscript questionnaires and found they were accurate, too. That fact was less surprising than it seemed, because draftees had been given the option not to fill out the survey if they didn't want to reveal their drug use at all.

With a bit of luck, Andréasson had found every researcher's dream. He had a large database that contained not just the key variable he needed but lots of secondary data too. Plus, another database that exactly captured the outcome at issue. All that was left was to compare the two.

So, he did, running the numbers to see whether conscripts who used cannabis before 1970 — ever, once in a while, or frequently — had developed schizophrenia by 1983.

Wow. That was Andréasson's first reaction when he saw the results.

Use of cannabis was strongly correlated with schizophrenia. And the risk was dose-related. In all, the questionnaires covered 45,570 conscripts. By 1983, 246 of them had been diagnosed with schizophrenia, or 0.54 percent. That figure was relatively low by international standards, reflecting the fact that Sweden set a high bar for the diagnosis.

Though cannabis use was rising in Sweden in the late 1960s, it was still relatively low. Only 4,290 conscripts had used the drug even once. They accounted for 49 cases of schizophrenia — a risk of 1.16 percent. Put another way, smoking even once more than doubled the risk.

But it was the risk in the heavier users that really jumped at Andréasson. Of the 752 conscripts who said they'd smoked fifty times or more, 21 later developed schizophrenia, a 2.8 percent risk — six times as high as people who had never smoked.

"We had a hypothesis that cannabis was a contributor to psychiatric disorder," Andréasson said. "But this was very much more powerful than we had expected."

The next step was trickier. Andréasson had to check to make sure the results weren't confounded. In other words, he had to check that the association that seemed to stem from cannabis didn't actually come from some other factor.

Confounding sounds complicated, but a hypothetical example may help explain it. Say, researchers find that people who buy air fresheners get lung cancer more often than those who don't. Uh-oh! Febreze causes cancer. Procter & Gamble's in trouble! Well, maybe not. Before those researchers blame air fresheners, they'd better figure out whether the people who buy them are also cigarette smokers. Because if they are, then fresheners don't cause cancer — those are just two things you get if you smoke.

In the case of schizophrenia and the Swedish conscripts, Andréasson knew several factors resulted in higher odds of schizophrenia — most important, a family history of mental illness. He had to adjust for those risks, along with other factors that might plausibly cause the disease, such as other drug use.

Andréasson knew most conscripts who developed schizophrenia were unlikely to have only cannabis use and no other risk factors. Some might have a family history of mental illness. Others had other risks. Each adjustment might reduce the strength of the statistical link that he had found. But he had to check all the potential confounding variables he could imagine. Otherwise the initial finding hardly mattered.

Fortunately for Andréasson, the huge size of the database — and the strength of the initial finding — worked in his favor. "Even when we considered all these background factors, we still saw the risk," he said. Use of cannabis more than ten times raised the risk of developing schizophrenia by 2.3

times even when Andréasson accounted for eleven different confounding factors. That adjusted risk wasn't quite as high as the "raw" figure — but it was still big.

Andréasson wrote up the findings and submitted the paper to the *Lancet,* the prestigious British medical journal. He highlighted the sixfold risk increase among heavy cannabis users. "Persistence of the association after allowance for other psychiatric illness and social background indicated that cannabis is an independent risk factor for schizophrenia," he wrote.

He expected he wouldn't hear anything for months. Winning publication in a top medical journal is very competitive. Many researchers spend their entire careers hoping to place a single article somewhere like the *Lancet.* Instead, the journal's editor wrote back almost immediately to say he wanted to run the paper as soon as possible.

"I was a young investigator," Andréasson said. "I had no experience with being treated with that kind of interest."

The *Lancet* published the paper, "Cannabis and Schizophrenia: A Longitudinal Study of Swedish Conscripts," on December 26, 1987. For the first time, a researcher had moved past case reports to demonstrate an actual statistical link between marijuana and schizophrenia.

The fact that risk increased with use was especially important. A core principle of epidemiology is that if *X* causes *Y*, then more *X* should cause more *Y*, exactly as Andréasson's data showed. "The more you used, the more risk you had," he said.

Later, Andréasson conducted a follow-up study to examine whether people who developed schizophrenia after smoking were different than schizophrenic patients who had not smoked. He found that smokers tended to be relatively high-functioning before their illness, while nonsmokers had been troubled from a much younger age — a more classic presentation of schizophrenia.

Based on his data and later findings, Andréasson says he believes that cannabis is responsible for between 10 percent and 15 percent of schizophrenia cases. Few people develop schizophrenia solely because of smoking, he thinks. But many who would not have become sick do so because marijuana pushes their vulnerable brains over the edge.

"Without cannabis, fewer people would develop the disorder," he says.

Andréasson hardly has rose-colored glasses about alcohol. He authored another paper based on the conscript data showing that even light drinking increased death rates. He is chairman of the Alcohol Policy Forum, a nonprofit group that helps craft Sweden's restrictive alcohol laws. But Andréasson believes that cannabis is significantly more dangerous. If people used marijuana as much as they drank, "we would see an enormous amount of morbidity from cannabis," he says.

The *Lancet* paper generated immediate interest. In the pre-internet era, many researchers wrote Andréasson about the findings. He even recalls an imprisoned child molester writing to ask if marijuana could have caused his behavior. In the thirty years since, other scientific studies have cited the article more than a thousand times, a huge number for any academic paper.

But the paper didn't end the argument on whether marijuana caused mental illness. In fact, as the 1980s came to a close, the debate was only beginning.

In the United States, so was an ultimately successful attempt to rebrand marijuana — a drug used as an intoxicant for thousands of years — as medicine.

FIVE:
MEDICAL MARIJUANA WINS

I have a confession.

I like Ethan Nadelmann.

For almost seventeen years, Nadelmann was the executive director of the Drug Policy Alliance, which advocates for cannabis legalization and reduced penalties on other drugs. He retired in April 2017, after demolishing his opponents, at least on the marijuana front.

Nadelmann didn't join the legalization movement to get rich — or high. He lives in a modest one-bedroom apartment with a view of an airshaft on Manhattan's Upper West Side. By his own account, he uses cannabis a couple of times a week. (He has a little stash of THC-infused chocolates in his dresser. He politely offered me one after our last interview. I politely declined.)

Nadelmann's tried most other drugs, too. Given his position, he felt almost a responsibility to understand their psychoactive and addictive qualities firsthand, he says. But Nadelmann never fell in love with drug culture or hedonism in general. A divorcé with one grown daughter, he's spent the last two decades in a cross-country relationship with Marsha Rosenbaum, another Drug Policy Alliance wonk. Keith Stroup's biggest backer was Hugh Hefner. Nadelmann's was George Soros, who has donated tens of millions of dollars to support legalized cannabis.

Born in 1957, Nadelmann grew up in Westchester County, north of New York City. He came of age during the first wave of marijuana legalization and went to college at McGill, in Montreal, before transferring to Harvard. He graduated in 1979 and entered a joint law-PhD program, also at Harvard. He planned to specialize in international law, with a focus on the Middle East. But the drug war grabbed his interest.

By 1981, Ronald Reagan had taken the White House. Cannabis use was declining, but cocaine use was still rising, thanks in part to falling prices. In a 1982 survey, 9 percent of men aged 18 to 25 said they had used cocaine in the last month. Abuse, addiction, and overdose followed. In response, the Reagan Administration pressed to destroy coca plants in the highland jungles of South America and block traffickers as they moved cocaine north. The administration was internationalizing the American drug war, trying to block supply at the source.

Nadelmann decided to write his PhD thesis about that effort. He focused on the way the State Department and Drug Enforcement Administration worked with foreign law enforcement agencies. He received surprising cooperation from the DEA, which hired him as a consultant to write a classified report about its practices.

Just as Nadelmann was seeing the drug war from the inside, crack took off — first in New York, Miami, and Los Angeles, then everywhere. Crack is cocaine that's been cooked with baking soda and water into a smokable pellet. Inhaling its fumes through a glass pipe produces a brief, intense euphoria. A journalist who smoked it described it in *The New Republic* as offering "the head rush of marijuana . . . with the clarity induced by a noseful of powder cocaine." A single small "rock" of crack cost only $5 or $10, making it cheap enough for poor people to try. Crack was an immediate hit, in the worst way. Its spread provoked a surge in violence caused both by the drug itself and turf battles between dealers.

Crime in the United States had been rising for decades, but crack supercharged it. In 1983, the United States had 1.25 million murders, assaults, and robberies — a rate of 538 violent crimes per 100,000 people, far higher than that of other rich countries. By 1991, the rate rose another 40 percent, to 1.9 million violent crimes. Almost 25,000 people were murdered that year, the highest total ever recorded in United States, nearly half the number of American soldiers who died in the entire Vietnam War. New York City alone had 2,154 killings.

Meanwhile, the AIDS epidemic was spreading. Along with gay men, heroin users were its main victims. But the Reagan White House would hardly acknowledge that AIDS existed, much less try to prevent it by giving addicts clean needles as AIDS activists wanted.

To Nadelmann, the explosion in crack-related violence, the spread of heroin-fueled HIV, and the hundreds of thousands of marijuana arrests every year all proved the same point: the American war on drugs was an insane mistake. He remembers telling two hundred intelligence analysts at a conference at Bolling Air Force Base in Washington, DC, in June 1987 that prohibition would inevitably end in failure. "I was nearly booed off the stage," he said.

In April 1988, he went public with his concerns in a *Foreign Policy* magazine article, "U.S. Drug Policy: A Bad Export." The next year, he wrote in the journal *Science* that the United States should consider legalization.

But Nadelmann was swimming upstream — not just on the issues of heroin and cocaine, but cannabis, too. NORML had never recovered from its collapse, and Republicans made mincemeat of Democrats who suggested that penalties for drug trafficking or dealing were tough enough already. The aggressive policies continued under George H. W. Bush, who became president in 1989. "The drug war [was] just going crazy," Nadelmann recalls. "It was like McCarthyism on steroids."

By then, Nadelmann was a professor at Princeton University. In the summer of 1992, Soros asked him to lunch. Already a billionaire investor, Soros would soon become famous for "breaking" the British pound — and in the process making a $1 billion profit. Soros had supported anti-Communist movements in Eastern Europe and the Soviet Union. Now that the Soviet Union had fallen, he wanted to expand his "open society" efforts to the West. He thought liberalizing drug policy might be a good place to start.

At lunch, Nadelmann sketched out a three-part strategy: decriminalizing marijuana, reducing penalties for other drugs, and increasing access to needles and drug treatment. While the media focuses on his role in marijuana legalization, he considered all three equally important, he says. "It's always about ending the broader drug war."

Soros liked Nadelmann's vision. In 1994, with Soros's backing, Nadelmann started the Lindesmith Center, named after Alfred Lindesmith, a sociologist who questioned whether drugs were as addictive as they seemed. Nadelmann also toned down his public rhetoric about legalizing drugs. (In 1993, he had said he hoped that within a few years "the right to possess and consume drugs may be as powerfully and as widely understood as the other rights of Americans.")

The crime wave in the United States had just crested. Drug arrests were still rising. In 1992, Bill Clinton had beaten George H. W. Bush to become the first Democratic president since Carter. But Clinton had won in part by making sure the Republicans couldn't portray him as weak on crime. In January 1992, as governor of

Arkansas, he'd famously supported the execution of a mentally impaired inmate named Ricky Ray Rector.

Nadelmann prepared to dig in for a long fight.

Then Proposition 215 took off from San Francisco and landed in his lap.

Prop 215 was the first medical marijuana initiative. It offered California voters the chance to change the state's laws so that anyone 18 or older could use marijuana with a physician's authorization. Initiatives are democracy at its most pure. Voters vote yes or no on them directly. They don't exist on the national level, only in some states. California is among the states where they are most frequently used.

The 1970s wave of marijuana decriminalization hadn't made much of the notion of marijuana as medicine. In *Marihuana Reconsidered,* Lester Grinspoon devoted only one thirteen-page chapter to the idea. But studies in the 1980s showed cannabis might help epilepsy and chemotherapy-related nausea. The studies were mostly small — more hypothesis generating than hypothesis testing. Still, they raised the question of whether marijuana might have medicinal uses.

Then AIDS activists in San Francisco began using marijuana to treat AIDS-related wasting. Ultimately, clinical trials would show cannabis was at best marginally helpful for the syndrome, which largely disappeared anyway after pharmaceutical companies introduced effective anti-HIV medicines. But at the time, activists said denying patients the chance to smoke as they were dying of AIDS was unfair and inhumane. They didn't want to legalize marijuana for recreational use, only medical purposes, they said.

The argument gained traction, especially in Northern California, one of the epicenters of the AIDS epidemic — and of cannabis use. But Nadelmann was reluctant to push a ballot initiative with uncertain prospects. A down vote would add to the narrative that marijuana was unpopular and should remain prohibited.

Still, Prop 215's backers were aggressive, so Nadelmann paid for a private statewide poll to see if the initiative had a chance statewide. To his surprise, it did. He brought the results to Soros. At the time, Soros didn't favor fully legalized marijuana, Nadelmann says. But Soros did like the idea of medical marijuana. He spent $550,000 to back the initiative.

Peter Lewis, the billionaire chairman of Progressive Insurance, and George Zimmer, the founder of Men's Wearhouse, together added another $760,000, at Nadelmann's urging. (While Soros was interested in drug reform for ideological reasons, marijuana was a personal issue for Lewis and Zimmer, who were regular smokers.) The three men accounted for almost two-thirds of the $2 million of the financing behind the initiative.

And on November 5, 1996, as Clinton swept to his second presidential term, Prop 215 won approval in California — clearing the way for medical marijuana in the state, and ultimately across the country.

The long-term importance of Prop 215 is hard to overstate. It spurred a chicken-and-egg reevaluation of marijuana's risks. In their wisdom, more than five million California voters had declared marijuana medicine. It couldn't be medicine if it was dangerous, could it? And it couldn't be dangerous if it was medicine, could it?

Marijuana's late-1970s association with cocaine had destroyed the legalization movement. The rebranding of cannabis as medicine helped undo that link. Plus, by 1990, cocaine use was declining sharply. Firsthand experience with the drug's dangers had turned Americans away from it. For the first time in a decade, cannabis advocates could put daylight between the two drugs.

The cocaine epidemic changed the dynamics around marijuana in a second, more subtle way. In the late 1970s, parents groups had proved a surprisingly effective counterweight to the cannabis lobby. They'd begun as volunteer organizations for parents upset about marijuana's effects on their children. But after Reagan became president, they became politicized. As the federal government increased spending on antidrug efforts, it wanted more control of the groups. And Nancy Reagan saw antidrug campaigns as a way to improve her image.

By the mid-1980s, "Just Say No," Nancy Reagan's pet phrase, had become the movement's motto. In 1987, her staff forced the nonprofit foundation behind Just Say No to accept a Procter & Gamble marketing executive as its director. The next year, the company sent 48 million homes a Just Say No pledge card — plus coupons for discounts on P&G products.

The corporate takeover hurt the legitimacy of the antidrug movement, while the rise of crack made parents groups seem out of touch. They came off as suburban Republicans hyperfocused on marijuana at a time when smokable cocaine was ravaging inner cities. The effect was to hollow out the ground-level opposition to cannabis, opening the way for Nadelmann and the next generation of advocates.

But for a while, the antimarijuana campaign still had momentum. Cannabis use plunged through the 1980s. By 1991, only one in four high school seniors said they had ever tried the drug, down from one in two in 1979. The number of Americans of any age who reported having used marijuana in the last year bottomed at 17 million in 1992, down from 33 million in 1979.

Yet arrests for marijuana, which had fallen along with use during the 1980s, suddenly began to rise. After bottoming at 290,000 in 1991, they reached 734,000 by 2000. The increase occurred mostly in arrests for possession rather than sale — users rather than dealers.

Several factors drove the crackdown. Police forces became aggressive about targeting minor crimes. They were following the "broken windows" theory, which held that failing to check low-level lawbreaking created an impression of disorder and allowed more serious crimes to flourish. In addition, police officers simply had more time to go after marijuana smokers. The number of officers in the United States rose by more than 100,000 during the decade, a nearly 20 percent increase, even as the crack epidemic waned.

"Police are now taking opportunities to make more marijuana arrests than they were when they were focused on crack cocaine," a criminology professor told the *Washington Post* in 2005.

The arrests rarely led to jail time, and almost never for simple possession. A 2005 paper from a liberal group called the Sentencing Project found that despite the huge number of arrests, fewer than 28,000 people in 2003 were incarcerated in federal or state prisons for marijuana offenses. Another 4,600 were held in county jails, for a total of 32,500 prisoners, out of almost 2.1 million nationally.

Many of those prisoners were traffickers who had moved pounds or even tons of marijuana. Even then, sentences could be surprisingly short. In 1994, for example, Vincent Capece was caught helping to smuggle $17 million of marijuana across the United States. Though he already had a record of drug offenses, he received a thirty-three-month sentence.

Even so, the arrests became a political issue. Civil libertarians and liberal groups focused on the fact that African Americans were arrested two to three times as often as whites, though the two groups had similar rates of marijuana use. (The groups skimmed over the fact that "similar" didn't mean the same; federal surveys showed that African Americans used marijuana somewhat more than whites, and those black people who did use tended to be heavier smokers. A 2016 paper in the journal *Drug and Alcohol Dependence* that was based on federal surveys covering more than 340,000 people showed that black people were almost twice as likely to report marijuana abuse or dependence as whites.)

The arrest gap provided an important way for marijuana's strongest advocates — who were overwhelmingly white and liberal — to approach the black community. African American leaders had seen the damage that alcohol and tobacco did in inner cities. They feared reducing restrictions on cannabis would cause similar problems, and many saw it as a gateway drug.

Cannabis supporters argued the arrests were the real problem. In a 2004 report, NORML argued:

It doesn't matter that many people arrested for marijuana possession do not spend time in jail beyond the time required for processing and arraignment before a magistrate; what matters is that any person arrested by police for marijuana possession can be sentenced to the maximum penalty allowed by law . . . marijuana laws are subjectively enforced and prosecuted.

In other words, black teenagers passing a joint in Harlem might be arrested and jailed, while white kids hitting a bong in Central Park would only be warned. The difference was unfair and racist, the advocates said. The argument didn't convert older black leaders overnight, but it gained traction among younger ones.

The racial disparity in arrests mattered less at first to most white people. To win them over, marijuana supporters argued that the crackdown on marijuana wasted money and the time of police officers who should focus on violent crimes. In reality, spending on marijuana arrests and post-arrest processing made up only about $4 billion of the $110 billion that the United States spent on police and courts in 2001, according to the Sentencing Project paper.

Still, the legalizers had found an issue that resonated. After 2000, the overall crime rate continued its long decline. Yet marijuana arrests rose, peaking at 872,000 in 2007. The disconnect fueled a sense among voters that the war on marijuana had gone too far.

Meanwhile, advocates continued their slow work — writing opinion pieces, highlighting the cost and racial disparities of the drug war, and offering grants to local pro-cannabis organizations. In July 2000, Nadelmann merged the Lindesmith Center with the Drug Policy Foundation — a Washington-based reform organization. The new group was called the Drug Policy Alliance. Soros would be its most important backer. Ultimately, he gave more than $100 million to the DPA and a related group that funded medical marijuana and legalization ballot initiatives. By 2010, he supported full legalization, and he wrote an opinion piece saying so in the *Wall Street Journal.*

Soros declined my request for an interview, but a spokeswoman for his Open Society Initiative, his philanthropic arm, wrote:

George Soros has been committed to drug policy reform since the early-1990s. He has seen how prohibitionist policies have disproportionally harmed the most marginalized populations and failed to protect society's most vulnerable people.

Nadelmann and Soros were not alone in their efforts.

In January 1995, a 25-year-old named Rob Kampia started the Marijuana Policy Project. As its name suggested, the MPP focused solely on cannabis. While Nadelmann saw the drug war as an intellectual and moral failure, the issue was more personal for Kampia. He had served ninety days in jail after being caught growing plants as an undergraduate at Penn State.

Like the original legalizers, Kampia liked to party, though he says alcohol was his drug of choice. (In 2010, the *Washington City Paper* published an article called "The Breast Massage Will Happen," a scathing investigation into Kampia's sexual harassment of MPP staffers.)

Whatever his personal demons, Kampia's single-minded focus on marijuana attracted the interest of Peter Lewis. "Peter's legalization mission was exactly the same as mine," Kampia told me. "It was to regulate marijuana like alcohol in the United States." Lewis cared less about Nadelmann's other drug-related projects, and the two men didn't particularly get along. So, Lewis backed MPP instead of the DPA. Before his death in November 2013 Lewis gave MPP more than $40 million to fund medical

141

marijuana and legalization initiatives, Kampia says.

Kampia was less guarded than Nadelmann, more willing to make aggressive claims about marijuana's medicinal properties. "If I had children, I would actually encourage them to use marijuana not just as a substitute for alcohol but because it has certain anticancer properties," he told me. Some legalizers would accept or even prefer a tightly regulated marijuana market, with high taxes, state-owned dispensaries with limited hours, or both. Kampia favors a fully free market, with low costs and wide availability. "You want marijuana to be significantly more available than alcohol or pills."

Still, Kampia and Nadelmann were colleagues more than rivals. Rather than competing to lead medical marijuana ballot initiatives, they divided them up by state. Each group led more than a dozen successful initiatives, helping draft the exact ballot language, fund-raising and gathering signatures, and paying for ads and campaign events.

Kampia always saw medical initiatives as a step to legalization. "[Only] six percent of all marijuana users use it for medical purposes," he said. "Medical marijuana is a way of protecting a subset of society from arrest."

Even more than the rise in arrests, medical marijuana had traction as an issue for advocates. Through the 1990s, Gallup polls showed that about only 25 percent of Americans favored legalizing marijuana. That figure perked up slightly in 1999, to 29 percent — while 69 percent opposed legalization.

But when it came to medical marijuana, Gallup found the numbers were reversed: 73 percent of Americans in 1999 favored "making marijuana legally available for doctors to prescribe in order to reduce pain and suffering." Only 25 percent opposed the idea.

By 2000, Alaska, Colorado, Oregon, Nevada, and Washington had all followed California and okayed medical marijuana. The idea appealed to Americans' sense of compassion; if marijuana could help sick people, why shouldn't they have it?

Yet the very wording of the Gallup question suggested the confusion around the issue. Even now, doctors cannot prescribe marijuana, because the FDA has never approved cannabis to treat any medical condition. Marijuana simply isn't a prescription drug in the way that physicians use the term. In modern medicine, a drug is usually a single chemical compound, like aspirin, taken as a pill or as an injection. (These days, some drugs are "biologics," complex molecules grown from specially engineered cells. But those biologics have even less in common with marijuana than ordinary chemical pharmaceuticals do.)

On the other hand, cannabis is a plant that contains many different chemicals, some of which work at cross purposes, like THC and CBD. Further, different strains have different levels of cannabinoids, so they can't be easily compared. Marijuana can be cooked and eaten or smoked in a cigarette — a method of use that the FDA could never condone. It can also be inhaled through a vaporizer as nearly pure THC.

The FDA generally approves pharmaceuticals only after years of closely controlled clinical trials. Doctors prescribe them at a set dose to treat a particular disease: take antibiotics for your sore throat for a week. Even drugs meant as long-term treatments, like medicines for diabetes, require patients to get new prescriptions when they finish their supply.

In contrast, medical marijuana laws allowed doctors to authorize patients to use cannabis for many different diseases, including nebulous conditions like insomnia or anxiety. (California's law allowed doctors to recommend it for any medical condition they saw fit.) Those authorizations lasted a year, and once a patient received one, he could use it to buy cannabis anytime he wished, for any reason.

In selling Prop 215 and later ballot initiatives, advocates promoted the idea that medical marijuana would be used *as medicine*. Posters featured a green leaf over a red cross, and slogans like "You've just been told you have terminal cancer. Now the bad news. Your medicine is illegal."

As the *Los Angeles Times* wrote in November 1996:

> The human face of Proposition 215, the medical marijuana initiative on Tuesday's ballot, is benign and sympathetic. It's right there in the backers' TV commercials: A breast cancer survivor who uses marijuana to ease nausea, a doctor who prescribes it to ailing patients, the widow of a cancer patient who used marijuana.

Mary Jane Rathbun — yes, Mary Jane was her real name — was the campaign's most prominent face. Rathbun had become known in San Francisco for the marijuana-

145

laced brownies that she cooked for AIDS patients. In July 1992, sheriff's deputies in Sonoma County, north of San Francisco, arrested her as she mixed marijuana into brownie batter. The charges were later dropped, but the arrest made "Brownie Mary" a celebrity across the state.

Spokespeople like Brownie Mary promoted the idea that medical marijuana would be used by genuinely sick people after careful discussions with their doctors. The reality was different. Most physicians didn't want to write medical marijuana authorizations, for both medical and legal reasons. The Drug Enforcement Administration initially tried to stop physicians from writing them at all, leading marijuana advocates to sue. After a 2002 decision against the government in the federal appeals court that covered California, the DEA backed off. Still, the issue was murky.

Aside from the potential legal jeopardy, many doctors thought medical marijuana was a bad idea. After seeing the dangers of tobacco, they didn't want to encourage smoking. Many knew the scientific evidence for using cannabis was weak. And doctors tend to be conservative when it comes to unproven treatments; the cardinal rule of medicine is first, do no harm.

As a result, a relative handful of cannabis-friendly doctors wrote most authorizations. California has more than 100,000 physicians; in 2011, NORML's list of doctors willing to write authorizations included about 1,500 names.

For the so-called pot doctors, medical marijuana cards became a volume business. At first, receiving an authorization in California cost $100 to $200 and required a serious consultation. But prices and standards dropped over time. Meanwhile, seriously ill people who wanted to discuss marijuana with their own doctors couldn't always do so. A 2010 article in *Mother Jones* highlighted the absurdity:

Recently, my wife and I had a contest. She'd ask her rheumatologist if he would write her a prescription for medical marijuana to treat her arthritis. I'd go online, find a doc, and see if I could get pot prescribed for a vague, undocumented medical problem. Then we'd see who'd be the first to join the ranks of California's 500,000 medical marijuana users.

After a $70, ninety-second "examination" in San Francisco with a "stooped, white-haired man in a rumpled pullover — the

147

doctor," the writer had his authorization. Meanwhile, his wife's rheumatologist said he couldn't help and referred her to her general practitioner, who also refused:

"I very rarely write letters for medical marijuana, and then it's only for advanced cancer," the doc explained. "I am not willing to write a letter for a relatively healthy 34-year-old."

Later, the *Mother Jones* writer found his way to the International Cannabis and Hemp Expo:

My medical marijuana card got me into a "patient consumption area" staffed by busty women in tight-fitting nurse outfits . . . As the refrain of "We Gotta Get High" hit the speaker, an employee of a San Jose–based dispensary wearing a nametag that said "Dr. Herb Smoker, MD" offered me a hit.

California didn't keep a mandatory registry of its patients, but surveys showed they were mostly white, under 45, and had been regular cannabis users before getting a medical card. Pain was a far more frequent reason for authorization than cancer or other serious illnesses. By 2014, some physicians charged as little as $30 for an authorization. Even medical marijuana supporters complained that the process was a joke.

The situation was similar elsewhere. In Oregon, which kept detailed data on authorizations, 10 of the state's 10,000 physicians accounted for 76 percent of all the authorizations written during the first decade of the program. One accounted for more than 35 percent.

At least in California and Oregon, patients had to see an actual physician for an authorization. Other states had even looser rules. The most stunning example was Arizona, where "naturopaths" could also write authorizations. Though they call themselves doctors, naturopaths do not attend regular medical schools or complete residencies in hospitals. They cannot practice surgery. Most states do not allow them to prescribe drugs.

Like Oregon, Arizona kept detailed statistics on which doctors wrote prescriptions (at least through the fiscal year ended June 30, 2015). During that year, about 78,000 Arizona residents received medical marijuana cards.

In 2015, Arizona had 30 times as many medical doctors as naturopaths. But the naturopaths accounted for nearly all the authorizations. The 23 busiest wrote 60 percent of all the authorizations in Arizona. Meanwhile, 98 percent of physicians didn't write a single authorization.

Despite the obvious loopholes it provided for recreational use, the medicalization of marijuana proved the crucial bridge to full legalization.

Not because the number of people authorized to use medical cannabis has ever been particularly high. The registries show that it is less than 1 percent of the population in most medical marijuana states, and more than 3 percent in only one state, Maine.

But medical legalization created a community of dispensaries and growers with a financial interest in full legalization. And it produced a stalemate between state and federal laws that allowed that community to flourish. Neither George W. Bush or Barack Obama wanted the spectacle of drug agents raiding medical marijuana dispensaries and dragging "budtenders" out in handcuffs.

Meanwhile, the backdoor protection the authorizations offered for recreational use increased pressure on voters in medical states to take the last step. With some justification, proponents of full legalization argued that dropping the fig leaf would result in better regulation and higher taxes.

Even in states that hadn't passed medical marijuana laws, everyone heard the same chorus: *marijuana is medicine, marijuana is medicine, marijuana is medicine.* No matter that the medical claims far outstripped the available evidence, and that when good studies were conducted, they were almost universally disappointing.

You might not be shocked to learn that Rob Kampia is wrong about cannabis and cancer, according to the National Academy of Medicine. In its 2017 report, NAM found essentially no evidence that cannabis or cannabinoids can help cancer of any kind. Worse, it found some evidence that cannabis use is associated with testicular cancer — and that mothers who smoke are more likely to have children who develop leukemias and brain cancer.

But it's not just cancer.

The National Academy's report also found no evidence that cannabis is useful for a whole alphabet of diseases it's supposed to help: dementia, epilepsy, glaucoma, irritable bowel syndrome, ALS (amyotrophic lateral sclerosis, or Lou Gehrig's disease), or Parkinson's disease. It found almost no evidence that marijuana can treat anxiety or posttraumatic stress disorder — and some evidence that the drug worsens those conditions.

The only conditions cannabis or cannabinoids have been proven to treat are chemotherapy-associated nausea and spastic muscles associated with multiple sclerosis, the report said. (Since the report appeared, CBD, the nonintoxicating compound in marijuana, has been shown to treat seizures associated with two rare forms of epilepsy, and the FDA has approved it for that condition.)

Smoking cannabis also seems to produce moderate pain relief. But the pain studies don't usually compare the degree of relief to standard pain relievers like ibuprofen, only to a placebo. More recently, a 1,500-patient, four-year study in Australia threw doubt on that finding, too.

Cannabis's general uselessness as medicine shouldn't surprise anyone who thinks through the issue. The human body is incredibly complicated. Hundreds of thousands of biomedical researchers worldwide spend their lives trying to figure out how diseases damage the body and how to stop them. Why would a single plant treat conditions as different as dementia, irritable bowel syndrome, and cancer? Even if it did, why would it treat them better than the compounds that scientists have discovered and refined over the last century? We don't pretend that garlic or nightshade cure diseases better than more modern medicines, so why do we do so for marijuana?

As Dr. David Gorski, a cancer surgeon and researcher, wrote on the blog *Science-Based Medicine* in 2015:

> I believe that marijuana should be legalized, regulated, and taxed, just like alcohol and tobacco. If marijuana is going to be approved for use as medicine rather than for recreational use, however, the standards of evidence it must meet should be no different than for any other drug, and for the vast majority of indications for which it's touted medical cannabis doesn't even come close to meeting that standard.

But aside from a few killjoys like Gorski, the same professional skeptics who insist guardian angels aren't watching us all, the idea of marijuana as a cure-all has no real opponents. At a time when Americans are hopelessly divided on issues from abortion to race relations, medical marijuana stands out for its nearly unanimous support. A 2017 national poll found that 94 percent of Americans supported "allowing adults to legally use marijuana for medical purposes if their doctor prescribes it."

Thirty states have now legalized medical marijuana, including Oklahoma, among the reddest of red states, in June 2018. Support for full recreational legalization remains weaker than for medical marijuana. But it too has climbed steadily, and now ranges over 60 percent in most polls, a figure high enough that politicians are paying attention. For the first time, some serious Democratic presidential hopefuls have called for legalization.

More surprisingly, John Boehner — a Republican who adamantly opposed legalization as Speaker of the House — announced in April 2018 that he had joined the board of a cannabis company, Acreage Holdings. "My thinking on cannabis has evolved," he said. (Boehner cannot be accused of being overly concerned about the risks of smoking, at least. He's a two-pack-a-day cigarette smoker. Paul Ryan, his successor as speaker, complained Boehner's office reeked of stale cigarettes after Ryan took it over.)

Even having a Republican in the White House probably won't turn the tide. Attorney General Jeff Sessions vehemently opposes cannabis. But his boss doesn't seem to care.

"Trump — on marijuana policy he's the best president who's ever existed on his stated intent," Kampia said. "He has not ever contradicted himself on the issue of having states determine their policies without federal interference."

Kampia thinks full national legalization is all but certain. Nadelmann agrees.

"I don't think it's really stoppable," he said. "The public support is so high . . . The broader question of issues like when and how marijuana is going to get legalized is not really an interesting question right now."

Instead, the debate will shift to issues like when and how the records of people who were arrested for marijuana should be expunged, Nadelmann said. The industry's commercial structure and attitude toward regulation will also be big issues. Nadelmann retired from DPA in part because he felt the next generation of advocates should lead those debates.

"The marijuana industry occupies a unique place in American history," Nadelmann said. "A movement driven by concerns for human rights, racial justice, and good public policy has resulted in the emergence of an industry that will be worth tens of billions of dollars a year."

For twenty-five years, marijuana legalizers have trounced their opponents by endlessly repeating two myths, that cannabis is effective medicine and that American prisons are filled with black people arrested for marijuana possession.

I'm sure advocates like Nadelmann and Kampia believe that marijuana is a relatively safe drug, illegal mainly because of American racism, and that the link between cannabis and mental illness is government propaganda to frighten kids. They've pounded that message over and over.

They've won and won and won.

They've been so busy winning they haven't noticed the proof they're wrong piling up.

■ ■ ■ ■

PART TWO:
PROOF

■ ■ ■ ■

SIX:
A ROUND-THE-WORLD
SEARCH FOR EVIDENCE

Sven Andréasson's 1987 paper in the *Lancet* moved the relationship between cannabis and mental illness out of the realm of *Reefer Madness.* Psychiatrists and researchers had to take seriously the possibility that marijuana could cause schizophrenia.

But possibility isn't fact. Andréasson had designed his study carefully. He had shown men who reported smoking cannabis developed the disease more often, and the more they smoked the higher the risk.

That association might mean the drug caused psychosis.

Then again, it might not. Other possibilities still existed. Skeptics offered four competing theories. In rough order of likelihood:

First, that the same genes that caused people to develop psychotic illnesses also encouraged them to use cannabis heavily. In that case, even though marijuana use

159

often preceded or accompanied schizophrenia, it would not be causal. People would become schizophrenic for genetic reasons whether or not they used.

Imagine looking at a highway at night in winter. The pavement seems clear, but it's actually covered with black ice. A dump truck scatters sand on the pavement. A few minutes later, a car drives past — and skids off.

The sand was put on the road before the accident, but did it cause the accident? Of course not. The ice did. But the ice is impossible to see. So, someone who relied only on the video to figure out what had happened might wrongly blame the sand. In reality, both the sand and the accident resulted from the ice.

In this analogy, the sand is cannabis use. The accident is schizophrenia. Our genes are the ice — the hidden fact that leads us to make an incorrect assumption about the events we can track.

The theory made intuitive sense. Schizophrenia was known to have a strong genetic component. Drug abuse also seemed to have some relationship to genes. But genetic science was in its infancy in 1987. Scientists had not yet decoded the human genome, much less discovered which mutations might be associated with schizophrenia or drug use.

As a result, no one at the time could prove or disprove the argument. To use Donald Rumsfeld's famous line, it was a "known unknown," a problem that could be outlined but not solved. (For a time, tobacco companies had tried the same argument about lung cancer, arguing that the same genes might both cause people to smoke cigarettes and raise their risk for lung cancer.)

Second, that although cannabis use seemed to cause schizophrenia, in fact the causation was reversed — the onset of the disease led to cannabis use. In its most extreme version, this theory held that cannabis might treat schizophrenia symptoms.

Doctors knew that many people who developed schizophrenia went through a slow decline before they suffered open breakdowns. As George Ewens had written in 1908: A gradual change of disposition; a loss of activity and energy, the patient becoming silly, shy, irritable, obstinate, and careless . . .

Psychiatrists now call that period the "prodrome." Prodromal patients are becoming ill but haven't yet snapped. They might hear voices from time to time or have intrusive thoughts and minor delusions —

161

everyone at school is laughing at me, or *I think my drink is spiked.* Their grades often slip. They may become disorganized or stop taking care of themselves. To cope, they begin to withdraw from friends and family.

But they are still well enough to understand that their thoughts are abnormal. They're anxious and depressed about their mental chaos. They smoke cannabis for the pleasure it produces or just to spend time with friends who are also smoking. Over time, as their psychosis progresses, they smoke more. Then they suffer an open break.

Because the heaviest use occurs just before the break, the drug seems to cause it. But according to this view, in fact smokers are using cannabis to try to control their symptoms. They're "self-medicating."

Andréasson had tried to account for this theory by excluding from his analysis recruits who were already suffering from schizophrenia when they were drafted. He only counted cases where recruits who were already smoking developed psychosis later. But Andréasson couldn't exclude the possibility that some recruits might have been suffering from hidden psychotic symptoms before the time of conscription — and possibly before they began to use marijuana.

Still, the self-medication theory faced big stumbling blocks. Psychiatrists knew that cannabis could cause temporary psychosis even in healthy people. They knew that many patients whose schizophrenia appeared under control suffered relapses if they used cannabis again. Andréasson also noted that even draftees with no evidence of depression or personality problems showed "an increased risk of schizophrenia with increasing cannabis consumption."

Researchers tried different arguments to square those facts with the self-medication theory. Maybe temporary cannabis psychosis didn't have anything to do with schizophrenia. Maybe people who already had developed schizophrenia started smoking again because they were relapsing and trying to control their symptoms with marijuana.

Those explanations weren't great. All in all, self-medication was less convincing than shared genetics as a hypothesis. But marijuana advocates would come to promote it. Unlike the genetic theory, it was easy to understand. Plus, it put a positive spin on the fact that so many people with mental illness smoked marijuana. See? Getting high is actually good for people with psychiatric disorders!

The third argument was that Andréasson's study had shown a falsely positive result by pure chance. Scientists say a clinical trial has proven its hypothesis if it has a "p-value" of 0.05 or less. In plain English, that number means that the trial has found a difference between two groups that has less than a 5 percent result of occurring by chance. But even at that standard, 1 trial in 20 may have a false finding. Andréasson's "crude" findings — before he accounted for confounders — were very strong, with p-values far below 0.05. But after he adjusted, he was on the edge of that 5 percent line. Maybe his trial was the 1 in 20 that had accidentally produced an invalid finding.

Like the genetic theory, this objection couldn't be answered immediately. But in the long run it would be the simplest to prove or disprove. If later studies on different populations failed to show a link, Andréasson's study would become less convincing. If they backed it up, his thesis would get stronger.

The fourth theory was that cannabis use was just a marker for other social or environmental problems that might cause schizophrenia. People whose parents were in prison, used drugs, or did poorly in school were more likely to use marijuana — and other drugs. Maybe those stressors or the other drugs were the real risks.

This theory was basically just confounders by another name, and Andréasson had gone out of his way to account for other variables. Plus, those other factors didn't seem to cause schizophrenia on their own, though they might worsen its course. It seemed more likely that cannabis stood apart from them. Still, the environmental theory couldn't yet be entirely discounted.

Psychiatrists and researchers batted around versions of those theories for fifteen years after Andréasson's paper without reaching definite conclusions. The need for more evidence — not just on the psychosis link, but on all of marijuana's potential risks and benefits — became clear in 1999. That year, the Institute of Medicine, the federally backed group that was later renamed the National Academy of Medicine, put out a report titled "Marijuana and Medicine: Assessing the Science Base."

The study was the last major effort to look at cannabis by the group before its 2017 paper. Reflecting the state of the science at the time, the 1999 paper is notably more positive than the later report, both in terms of marijuana's benefits and its risks.

"Except for the harms associated with smoking, the adverse effects of marijuana use are in the range of effects tolerated for other medicines," the report found. It recommended continued research into marijuana for many diseases.

In terms of negatives, the report focused on potential physical hazards from smoke and largely discounted other concerns. Only a few smokers became dependent on marijuana, withdrawal symptoms were "mild and short-lived," and no evidence proved that marijuana use led to harder drugs.

As for mental illness, the 1999 report hardly mentioned it. It said cannabis psychosis was almost always temporary and dealt with schizophrenia in a single paragraph, saying "The relationship between marijuana and schizophrenia is not well understood." It even suggested "the possibility that schizophrenics might obtain some symptomatic relief from moderate marijuana use."

Time and further research have not been kind to that theory. They have been even harsher on the report's view on prescription opiates, which is worth noting because it informed its findings on the potential positives of medical marijuana. The report lauded the late-1990s trend toward increased opiate prescribing:

> [Fears] that liberal use of opiates would result in many addicts . . . have been proven unfounded . . . Few people begin their drug addiction problems with misuse of drugs that have been prescribed for medical use . . . the diversion of medically prescribed opiates to the black market is not generally considered to be a major problem.

Six hundred thousand overdose deaths later in the United States, it's fair to say the report — and pro-opiate physicians more generally — underestimated the risks of encouraging opiate prescriptions and use.

The fact that scientists twenty years ago understood so little about cannabis and the brain didn't help. Research into what was becoming known as the endocannabinoid system was in its infancy. Only in 1988 had researchers discovered the CB1 receptor, the structure on brain cells that THC activated. The hippocampus, which helped form memories, and the amygdala, which helped govern emotion, memory, and fear, both had heavy concentrations of the receptors.

In 1992, scientists discovered ananda-mide, an "endocannabinoid," a chemical our own bodies produce to stimulate CB1 receptors. But researchers weren't sure exactly how anandamide interacted with dopamine and other neurotransmitters. Anandamide was hard to study, too. The stuff barely even existed permanently in brain cells or channels. It was produced as needed and then quickly destroyed.

Scientists also discovered that triggering CB1 receptors indirectly caused some dopamine release, although it was concentrated in a different part of the brain than the dopamine release that opiates caused. Still, the fact that THC could increase dopamine levels helped explain the high associated with marijuana. It also hinted at an answer for its link to psychosis.

But the difficulties of translating basic neuroscience research into the thought distortions of psychosis — the difficulties of turning brain into mind — meant that stronger proof would have to come from somewhere else.

A collaboration between researchers on opposite ends of the globe provided the next step.

Dunedin is a picturesque city of 120,000 on the southeast coast of New Zealand's

South Island — a rock in the Pacific Ocean, a long way from anywhere. In the late 1960s, a Dunedin pediatrician named Patricia Buckfield created a database of all the babies born in the Queen Mary Hospital, the city's obstetric center. Buckfield planned to track the relationship between prenatal problems and later health complications.

In 1971, Phil Silva, a schoolteacher-turned-psychologist, joined Buckfield's research, which initially focused on just 250 kids. Silva noticed that a lot of those children had developmental problems their family pediatricians had not diagnosed. He pushed for a larger study that would include all the babies born between April 1972 and March 1973 whose families still lived in Dunedin in 1975. The potential pool included 1,139 children. Most of their parents — covering 1,037 children in all — agreed to participate in what became known as the Dunedin Multidisciplinary Health and Development Study.

At first, Silva expected the study would include only a single assessment when the children were three. "The resources for the Study were scarce," he wrote in a 1996 book about the project. Aside from a part-time secretary, Silva mostly relied on volunteers at first. They conducted assessments of the children in the Sunday school classroom of a local church. But Silva kept finding new funds to support and extend the project.

The kids were measured again at ages 5, 7, 9, 11, 13, 15, 18, and 21. Each time nearly all took part. By then, the study's value was obvious. Dunedin was not the largest study of its kind, but it was probably the most comprehensive in terms of tracking participants. The high participation rate was crucial. Long-term social science studies had the same dynamics as high school reunions — the most successful people were the most likely to come back.

But the Dunedin researchers went to great lengths to make sure the children and their families understood the value of the study. Only once, at age 13, did fewer than 90 percent take part. In later years the rate increased. The researchers got to know the participants well and promised confidentiality even for potentially criminal behavior such as drug use or violence. The New Zealand police didn't try to interfere. As a result, the Dunedin research truly described the entire group, for better or worse.

As the survey progressed, Silva added permanent staff and more researchers. On a trip to Los Angeles in the early 1980s, he met Terrie Moffitt, a psychology graduate student at the University of Southern California whose research focused on the reasons people became violent. Moffitt had broken her leg in a skydiving accident and was temporarily stuck in a wheelchair, so she and Silva had plenty of time to talk. In 1985, Moffitt joined the study — while simultaneously becoming an assistant professor at the University of Wisconsin. For the next several years, she split her time between Madison and Dunedin, a mere 8,700 miles apart.

By the mid-1990s, the Dunedin research had attracted international attention. A psychiatrist named Robin Murray was among those who noticed. A Scottish native, Murray has spent most of the last five decades researching and treating schizophrenia at the Institute of Psychiatry, Psychology & Neuroscience of King's College London.

Murray was born in 1944 in Glasgow, the son of teachers. He grew up in rural Scotland but came back to Glasgow for medical school. His interest in psychiatry took off after he spent a year living in a psychiatric hospital as a medical student. In exchange for free room and board, he had to examine the patients periodically. He found their damaged minds fascinating.

In 1972, he moved to London to begin his residency in psychiatry at "the Maudsley" — Maudsley Hospital, a campus of brick buildings in Denmark Hill, a low-income section of South London. Three years later he joined the Institute of Psychiatry, which shares the Maudsley's campus and is the largest research center for psychiatry and neuroscience in Europe.

Aside from a single year working at the NIMH (National Institute of Mental Health) in Maryland, Murray has remained in London ever since. In 2010, another professor joked that Murray's career was "a rare example of institutionalization being wholly positive for both the institution and the individual."

In the 1970s and 1980s, Murray focused on the genetic underpinnings of psychosis and the structural changes to the brain that schizophrenia seemed to cause — the core of American research. But over time, Murray grew to believe that psychosis resulted not just from genetics but from disturbances in infancy, childhood, and young adulthood. The fact that Denmark Hill was located near Brixton, a poor London neighborhood with high rates of cannabis use and schizophrenia, helped convince him. He became interested in the possibility of a link between cannabis and psychosis.

Other psychiatrists at the institute also wanted to investigate how environment and genetics might combine to cause mental illness. In 1994 King's College and a British government group created the Social, Genetic & Developmental Psychiatry Centre at the Institute of Psychiatry.

Meanwhile, in New Zealand, Phil Silva was nearing retirement. Terrie Moffitt had become the project's associate director. In 1995, Michael Rutter, a child psychiatrist at King's, convinced Moffitt to bring the Dunedin data to the new center, though London was 11,000 miles from the South Coast — an even longer haul than Madison.

By then, the Dunedin project had come a long way from its modest roots. Further assessments were conducted starting in 1998, when participants were 26, as well as when they turned 32, 38, and 45. The plan now is to continue the study through the lives of the participants. Secondary research will examine their children and even their grandchildren. The project will long outlast Silva, its founder, who retired in 2000. Silva is nearly 80 now and complained via email that he was "going deaf and losing vision fast. That is called ageing." Still, he had enough energy to take credit for his work: "I founded the world-renowned Dunedin study in the early '70s and directed it for 30 years. I taught the present director, Richie Poulton, most of what he knows, and Terrie Moffitt taught him the rest."

With Moffitt on board, Robin Murray looked for fresh ways to use the Dunedin data. He liked to encourage collaboration among young researchers. He put together Mary Cannon, an Irish psychiatrist and epidemiologist, with a Canadian psychologist named Louise Arseneault. (In fact, Arseneault had just written a paper based on the Dunedin data that examined risk factors for violence; more on that finding later.)

"Robin Murray said I should go meet with Louise Arseneault," Cannon told me. "I came from a psychosis background, and she was studying delinquent behavior in young people. We worked well together."

Murray encouraged Arseneault and Cannon to see what the Dunedin data revealed about cannabis and mental illness. "I remember having discussions with Robin Murray," Arseneault said. "We decided to explore the link between schizophrenia and cannabis."

In one way, Dunedin was not ideal for this work. With fewer than 1,000 participants in its age-26 pool, it was unlikely to generate more than ten full-blown schizophrenia cases. With such a small sample, even a strong marijuana-schizophrenia link wouldn't pass the 0.05 p-value test.

To increase the sample size, the researchers included people with a diagnosis of schizophreniform syndrome. Those were psychotic episodes that ended within six months and thus didn't quite reach full-blown schizophrenia. Though less severe than schizophrenia, schizophreniform syndrome was still a destructive illness.

But the Dunedin data offered advantages, too. New Zealand had high rates of cannabis use, so the dataset offered a large number of people who'd used the drug. More important, unlike almost any other studies, it had data on preteen, premarijuana-use symptoms of psychosis. A psychiatrist who interviewed the children when they were 11 had asked them about psychotic symptoms.

The age-11 data meant that Arseneault and Cannon could account for preexisting psychosis when they tried to find if cannabis use caused later psychotic disease. Plus, the data on marijuana use at age 15 had been collected when the participants were age 15, not years later. It didn't depend on the memories of participants, and researchers didn't have to reconstruct it afterward, when they already knew who had developed full-blown psychosis.

"You have such good data collected prospectively," Cannon says. "That's the most important thing — this data was collected without any bias."

Arseneault and Cannon ran the numbers. They knew of Andréasson's *Lancet* paper, but they weren't sure if they would have similar results, Arseneault says. "You never know what you're going to find."

What they found jumped at them.

People who had used cannabis at age 15 were more than 4 times as likely to develop schizophrenia or schizophreniform syndrome as those who never used. Even after accounting for those kids who had shown psychotic symptoms at age 11, the risk remained threefold higher.

"A fourfold increased risk was very big," Cannon says. When it came to psychosis and schizophrenia, she was used to seeing slight increases in risk — 10 percent or 20 percent.

With Arseneault as the lead author, they wrote a paper on their findings. "Using cannabis in adolescence increases the likelihood of experiencing symptoms of schizophrenia in adulthood," they reported. "Our findings agree with those of the Swedish study."

In what was becoming a trend, they submitted it to the *British Medical Journal* and the *Lancet,* but not the top American medical journals. The *BMJ* ran the paper in its November 23, 2002, edition, along with an update of the original Swedish paper and a third study from Australia that examined links between cannabis and depression.

Meanwhile, in a paper published a few months earlier, Dutch psychiatrists had reported that cannabis seemed to cause psychosis in some healthy adults. In 1996, the researchers randomly chose thousands of adults in the Netherlands. They asked the participants about cannabis use and interviewed them to see if they had any psychotic symptoms. The researchers followed up again after a year, and then after three years. They wound up interviewing more than four thousand people in all; more than 98 percent did not have a psychotic disorder.

Three years later, 7 out of 300 previously healthy adult marijuana smokers had developed psychosis or serious psychotic symptoms. Over the same period, only 3 of more than 3,600 people who did not smoke developed psychosis or serious psychotic symptoms.

Many people who used cannabis also used other drugs, the study found. But when the researchers adjusted for other drug use, the psychosis risk of cannabis users remained strong. The scientists estimated that cannabis use might be responsible for as much as half the serious psychosis in previously healthy adults.

Taken together, the Swedish, Dutch, and New Zealand studies provided powerful evidence linking cannabis to mental illness. In a *BMJ* editorial discussing them, two Australian psychiatrists wrote:

> Although the number of studies is small, these findings strengthen the argument that use of cannabis increases the risk of schizophrenia and depression, and they provide little support for the belief that the association between marijuana use and mental health problems is largely due to self-medication.

All three papers received plenty of scientific attention, especially the one by Arseneault and Cannon. Their paper has been cited more than 1,300 times since they published it, even more than Andréasson's 1987 paper.

Cannon, now a professor of psychiatric epidemiology in Ireland as well as a practicing psychiatrist, says she expected that the 2002 findings would have a big impact on public attitudes. After all, three sets of researchers in three different countries had come at the question of marijuana and psychosis from three different directions. They all had reached the same conclusion. Cannon expected that the consensus would move close to ending the debate.

But it didn't. Skeptics argued the Dunedin study was too small to be meaningful and that the Swedish data depended on self-reported cannabis use. Plus, the genetic objection remained unanswered.

"People were very polarized by this," Cannon said. "I thought the data was very clear, and people were saying this cannot be true, it cannot be causal . . . To me, it's just so blindingly obvious — we've found this incredibly robust effect, and it's been confirmed a number of times now."

In the United Kingdom, perhaps the best-known doubter was David Nutt, a brain researcher and member of a government commission that advised British lawmakers on the relative dangers of drugs. Britain classifies drugs as Class A, B, or C, depending on their dangers. Class A drugs, like heroin, carry the harshest consequences. Class B drugs have lesser penalties, though users and dealers can still face jail time, and Class C lesser still. When the *BMJ* published its research in 2002, Britain categorized cannabis as a Class B drug. But the government advisory committee had just recommended that it be moved to Class C.

For Britain, a move from B to C was the rough equivalent of decriminalization in the United States. Marijuana would still technically be illegal, but both police and users would know that it was viewed far less seriously than drugs like heroin. The committee stuck to its advice despite the new research. In 2004, Britain moved cannabis to Class C.

Yet, surprisingly, cannabis use did not increase in Britain after the reclassification — in part because of Robin Murray and the Institute of Psychiatry. The institute and genetics center eventually grew to 150 psychiatrists, neuroscientists, epidemiologists, graduate students, and other researchers. And Murray is at the heart of the institute, as I found when I traveled to London to see him and the place firsthand.

Now in his mid-seventies, Murray remains energetic, writing papers, treating patients, and traveling worldwide to conferences on mental illness. Even his personal life is inextricably interlinked with schizophrenia research; Marta Di Forti, Murray's second wife, also works at the institute, and they regularly collaborate. Over the years, Murray has helped train hundreds of young psychiatrists. Forty have become full professors. With his encouragement, many became interested in the cannabis-psychosis link:

- "Cannabis Use and Outcome of Recent Onset Psychosis," *European Psychiatry,* June 2005.
- "The Environment and Schizophrenia: The Role of Cannabis Use," *Schizophrenia Bulletin,* July 2005.
- "What Is the Mechanism Whereby Cannabis Use Increases Risk of Psychosis?" *Neurotoxicity Research,* June 2008.
- "The Acute Effects of Synthetic Intravenous Δ9-Tetrahydrocannbinol on Psychosis, Mood, and Cognitive Functioning," *Psychological Medicine,* October 2009.

Murray coauthored those papers and more than eighty others on cannabis and psychosis. Not all were pathbreaking. Some were small environmental studies that followed patients. Others were reviews of earlier research.

But even the secondary efforts kept British journalists and politicians aware of the issue. The institute's researchers had a big structural advantage. They worked in a neighborhood with lots of cannabis use and psychosis, yet not even five miles from the heart of London — England's business, government, and media center. They could reach news organizations easily, and they succeeded in getting their message out. In 2007, *The Independent,* a British newspaper that had endorsed cannabis decriminalization, reversed its view. In October 2008, the British government reclassified cannabis back to a Class B drug.

By then, David Nutt had become the British government's chief drug advisor. But the reclassification frustrated him, and he took some outlandish positions. In 2009, he wrote a paper called "Equasy: A Harmful Addiction," arguing that riding horses was much more dangerous than Ecstasy, an amphetamine derivative. If horse-riding was legal, Ecstasy should be, too, he wrote. The government fired him soon after.

In 2010, Nutt continued in the same vein with a paper claiming alcohol was more harmful than cocaine or even heroin. Alcohol does kill more people than heroin, because it is used so much more widely; about 70 percent of American adults drink at least once a year, and more than half at least once a month.

But even before the opiate epidemic, no one doubted that heroin would have catastrophic consequences if it were used as widely as alcohol. Large studies have shown that about one-third of people who use heroin even once become addicted and that opiate addicts die at 10 to 20 times the rate of nonusers. (For cocaine, the addiction rate seems to be in the 20 percent range, and addicts die at 4 or 5 times the rate of nonusers.)

Since then, Nutt, who remains a professor of neuropsychopharmacology at Imperial College London, has been involved in a quixotic effort to develop a product he calls "alcosynth," a replacement for alcohol. "The drinks industry knows that by 2050 alcohol will be gone," he told *The Independent* in 2016. "But they don't want to rush into it, because they're making so much money."

While Nutt chased synthetic alcohol, Robin Murray's reputation grew. In 2011, he received a knighthood — making him Sir Robin Murray, though after seeing his rumpled clothes, I had a difficult time imagining anyone calling him sir. He became the most highly cited schizophrenia researcher in Europe.

And the repeated warnings from King's College didn't just get media attention. They helped change the way Britain views cannabis.

In 2001, more than half of British adults favored legalization of cannabis, according to the British Social Attitudes Survey. By 2010, only about 1 in 3 did. Since then, the percentage has increased, but it remains below 50 percent. A 2016 survey of UK students showed that they associated cannabis strongly with mental health problems. A Twitter search for "cannabis psychosis" shows British teenagers and young adults discussing the issue as a serious risk.

Meanwhile, British cannabis use has plunged. From 2000 to 2005, more than 10 percent of adults and almost 30 percent of young adults used at least once a year, according to British government surveys. Now the figures are about 6 percent for adults and 17 percent for young adults.

Maybe the most telling proof of the effectiveness of Murray's efforts came in the jeers that British pro-cannabis campaigners launched against the Institute of Psychiatry. In 2015, CLEAR (Cannabis Law Reform), an advocacy group, complained on its website about the "anti-cannabis cult at King's College."

CLEAR trotted out the old argument that psychosis research has confused correlation and causation — as if scientists worldwide have not spent the generation since Sven Andréasson's paper teasing out cause and effect. "The team at King's College displays all the classic markers of a cult. It pursues a belief in cannabis as the 'devil's lettuce' as a quasi-religion . . . it endlessly repeats itself, its 'studies' and its presentation of them as proof," CLEAR wrote.

Three days later, CLEAR went further, implying without evidence that Murray and other researchers benefitted financially from their findings. "We simply cannot rely on these so-called eminent scientists to be honest about their work. They are in the gutter and they aren't looking at the stars, they are looking at their bank balances."

In fact, Murray has no financial interest in cannabis research. He has always been careful not to position himself explicitly against legalization. In 2009, in the wake of the classification controversy, he wrote in *The Guardian,* a British newspaper: "I care little whether cannabis is classified as a class B or class C drug. Fourteen-year-olds starting daily cannabis use do not agonise over its exact classification . . ." He simply wanted to educate people about the drug's mental health risks and build a consensus against teenage use, he said.

Still, Murray clearly doesn't favor legalization. When I asked him if he was surprised that so many American states had legalized, he gave me his only off-the-record answer, then added, "I've been surprised by the power of the business lobby for cannabis."

Seven:
An Unlikely Theory
Gains Traction

Robin Murray is right. The American marijuana industry is increasingly powerful and well-financed. As *USA Today* wrote in April 2018, cannabis investors have "built — largely unseen — a powerful network of businesses poised to take advantage of a more favorable federal climate. That industry already has woven itself into the fabric of states where pot is legal."

But the industry here also has a huge advantage in spreading its dubious messages about marijuana safety. The link between cannabis and psychosis isn't nearly as well known outside Britain — at least in part because the United States has no research center like the Institute of Psychiatry.

Of course, the United States has had hundreds, if not thousands, of scientists devoted to studying psychosis. Many are interested in marijuana. But they are scattered across the country. And some of the places best positioned to do marijuana-related work do none at all.

The most glaring example is at the University of Colorado, which has a schizophrenia research center at its Denver campus. Its chair is Dr. Robert Freedman, a respected psychiatrist who edited the *American Journal of Psychiatry* from 2006 through 2018. Considering that Colorado has among the highest rates of cannabis use anywhere, the center would seem to be in a unique position to study the drug's effects.

It has indeed focused on the relationship between smoking and schizophrenia.

Smoking cigarettes, that is.

For decades, Freedman has centered his research on whether nicotine-like drugs can help the cognitive symptoms of schizophrenia. The federal government has given him millions of dollars for studies.

Yes, treating the cognitive symptoms of schizophrenia is important. Yes, scientific research is about failure as well as success. Researchers can't know if their theories will work until they test them. But the fact that a schizophrenia research center in Colorado hasn't even looked at marijuana seems like an incredible missed opportunity.

The federal National Institute on Drug Abuse has a $1 billion annual budget. But for the last decade it has understandably focused on the opiate crisis. And because NIDA is a government agency, research it conducts or pays for — no matter how objective — can always be criticized as biased against marijuana.

In contrast, the Institute of Psychiatry can't be accused of having a structural bias against marijuana. It doesn't just work for the British government. Its researchers collaborate with pharmaceutical companies to research CBD and other cannabinoids for medical purposes. (A side note: Studies have shown CBD to be weakly effective in reducing some psychotic symptoms, leading to marijuana is good for schizophrenia stories from news outlets that should know better. In August 2017, a *Forbes* headline claimed that "Cannabis Shows Promise in Treating Schizophrenia." No, no, no. Once again, CBD isn't cannabis. It's one chemical in marijuana out of many. And unlike THC, CBD doesn't activate the CB1 brain receptor. Whether or not CBD helps psychosis has nothing to do with whether THC worsens it. Finally, it bears repeating that nearly all marijuana sold today contains high levels of THC and almost no CBD.)

Yet the trans-Atlantic knowledge gap has also exposed a structural difference between

Europe and the United States. American researchers often focus on the ways that mental illness affects the brain on the cellular level. They make careers of running neuroimaging studies examining the brains of people with psychosis. But decades of that work have so far produced no useful new drug treatments or reliable ways to predict who may develop schizophrenia. Research that links the brain changes that cannabinoids produce to psychotic symptoms is even more primitive.

"Brain research around cannabis is at a relatively novel stage," says Valentina Lorenzetti, a neuroscientist at Australian Catholic University who studies the way the drug affects brain cells and structure. "There isn't much strong evidence. We need so much more work."

British and European researchers are often more interested in the epidemiology behind mental illness — teasing out patterns among users. That work is less likely to lead to cures but often more useful for prevention. Epidemiologists realized that cigarette smoking caused lung cancer long before cancer researchers figured out exactly how the tars in tobacco damaged lung cells.

But new treatments are far sexier — and more profitable — than public health advice. Robert Freedman co-owns patents related to screening the nicotine receptor gene for schizophrenia-related mutations. He is listed on another patent for one of the nicotine-like drugs his center has studied. Did those financial interests encourage Freedman's obsession with nicotine at a time when marijuana use was exploding? Only he knows for sure.

So, while British psychiatrists pounded away on the cannabis-psychosis connection, American doctors ceded the field to legalizers. In Britain, Robin Murray was probably the most important voice on cannabis. In the United States, Ethan Nadelmann and Rob Kampia played that role, aided by journalists.

Americans heard little about marijuana's mental health risks and plenty about its benefits. And they listened. An annual survey of American high school students showed that in 2005, about 60 percent of seniors saw great harm in smoking marijuana regularly. By 2017, fewer than 30 percent of seniors felt that way. Adult surveys showed similar trends.

No surprise, after remaining roughly flat from 2000 through 2006, American marijuana use began rising in 2007. It hasn't stopped since.

In 2005, Americans and people in Britain used marijuana at roughly the same annual rates. By 2016, American adult rates had risen 50 percent, while British rates fell more than a third. That year, about 14 percent of American adults reported having used marijuana, more than double the British rate. American adults were more likely to have used cannabis in the last month than British adults were in the last year.

The legalization community likes to call the United States exceptional in its attitudes toward drugs, implying that Europe has a more civilized attitude toward marijuana. They're right. The United States is exceptional. But not because it's strict. The United States has the loosest laws and highest rates of cannabis use among any major countries. It also has the noisiest, most aggressive community of users.

The same Twitter search for "cannabis psychosis" that turns up British teenagers writing about psych wards finds Americans complaining about Big Pharma conspiracies to demonize their favorite weed. In Colorado, which has supplanted Northern California as the center of the modern American marijuana industry, the proselytizing is especially aggressive.

I saw and heard their attitudes for myself

last April, when I visited Colorado to see the "420" festivities. (Since the 1970s, smokers have used the term "420" to refer to marijuana. Many now treat April twentieth as a quasi-holiday.) In Colorado Springs, I stopped at a dispensary called Epic Remedy. "For heads by heads," its logo proclaimed.

It's worth noting that tolerance of THC rises far more quickly than alcohol tolerance does. Usually, 2.5 milligrams of THC are considered the equivalent of one drink. But regular marijuana users can use 100 milligrams or more daily, the equivalent of 40-plus drinks for a novice user, and still function.

The difference in tolerance probably occurs in part because cannabis is less physically toxic than alcohol, so in that way it is a sign of marijuana's safety. Still, it has a paradoxically negative effect. It means that heavy marijuana users make up a huge portion of overall cannabis use. In *Marijuana Legalization: What Everyone Needs to Know*, a 2016 book, three nonpartisan researchers explain that "normal marijuana use more closely resembles binge drinking than it does mere drinking." Only 10 percent of drinkers use alcohol every day. But about one-third of marijuana users smoke every day. Further, because use is so concentrated, heavy consumers of THC are even more important to cannabis companies than heavy drinkers are to alcohol companies. Thus, dispensaries and users wind up with a shared interest in keeping cannabis taxes low and playing down the effects of heavy use.

As I pulled out of the Epic Remedy parking lot that day in Colorado Springs, the afternoon hosts on KOA — a popular Denver news-talk station — were discussing a survey that showed 15 percent of people in the state had reported using marijuana on the job. Callers explained they smoked vapes, which can be odorless, for their entire shifts. I couldn't imagine a liquor store marketing itself as "For drunks by drunks," or callers to a radio show proudly explaining that they were nipping vodka all day at the office.

On KOA, the hosts pushed back against one particularly cannabis-happy caller, asking if he would be comfortable having a surgeon operate on him after smoking. Yes, the man responded, after coming up with a bizarre hypothetical scenario where the surgeon had operated all night on another patient and needed to sleep for a few hours before returning to the operating room. *I'd rather have him smoke and get to sleep naturally than take a sleeping pill,* he said.

Hearing the caller contort himself to justify a surgeon getting high was almost funny. It would have been, anyway, if it hadn't been so reminiscent of the newest strategy that advocates have used to promote their drug — calling marijuana a way to reduce opiate use, a theory breathtaking in its counterfactual audacity.

The belief that marijuana might somehow be a solution to the opiate epidemic took hold after October 2014. That month *JAMA Internal Medicine* published a paper claiming that states that legalized medical marijuana had a 25 percent reduction in opiate overdose deaths between 1999 and 2010 compared to those that didn't. The reduction was greatest immediately after legalization but persisted afterward, the paper found.

"Medical cannabis laws are associated with significantly lower state-level opioid overdose mortality rates," the paper's author, Dr. Marcus Bachhuber, reported. In 2010, the laws had resulted in 1,729 fewer deaths than expected, he wrote.

The finding has since become accepted wisdom. Other researchers have cited Bachhuber's paper more than 250 times. Marijuana companies advertise its findings as fact on electronic billboards in cannabis-legal states. In February 2018, Dr. Richard A. Friedman, a psychiatrist at Weill Cornell Medical College, wrote an opinion piece in the *New York Times* called "Marijuana Can Save Lives." Friedman pointed to the *JAMA* paper's findings to criticize Attorney General Sessions for enforcing federal laws against marijuana.

"Marijuana isn't a gateway drug to opioid addiction; it's a safer alternative to pain medicines. Mr. Sessions's vow to crack down on marijuana will only make the opioid epidemic worse," Friedman wrote. "If cannabis were actually a dangerous gateway drug, as the attorney general suggested, it would be very easy to see in the data. We would find that medical-marijuana laws increased opiate drug use and overdose deaths, when in fact just the opposite has happened."

Just the opposite?

Even at the time *JAMA* published Bachhuber's paper, its findings should have been viewed as dubious for a half-dozen reasons.

Many previous studies had shown marijuana use was connected to later heroin use. Researchers had found opiate addicts in methadone treatment relapsed more frequently if they used marijuana. Other studies showed adolescents who used marijuana were more likely to use heroin later, the so-called gateway theory Friedman mentioned.

Two of the most interesting studies looked at twins. A 2003 study that examined twins in Australia found that in cases where one twin used cannabis before 17 and the other did not, the twin who used was almost four times as likely to develop an opiate or cocaine use disorder. A 2006 study of twins in the Netherlands found even bigger risks from early use.

The twin studies naturally controlled for both genetics and upbringing — twins lived in the same house at the same time, and identical twins had the same genes. The gap "could not be explained by common familial risk factors, either genetic or environmental," the Netherlands researchers wrote.

Other researchers argued against the gateway theory, noting that plenty of people used marijuana without moving on to opiates, cocaine, or other drugs. But until Bachhuber, no serious researcher had suggested that marijuana use — whether called recreational or medicinal — might actually discourage other drug use.

Okay, but the *JAMA* paper focused on

medical marijuana. Maybe medical marijuana was different than recreational. Only it wasn't. The drug was the same, of course. And as you've already learned, most people who used medical marijuana had been recreational users and received authorizations from doctors who specialized in writing them.

Bachhuber's paper also showed a very strange time effect. Early medical marijuana programs needed years to accumulate significant numbers of patients. Smokers didn't want to join state registries before they were sure authorities wouldn't use the participation against them. Colorado's registry had only 94 patients during the first year of its program, in 2000. Until 2009, it never had more than five thousand patients. Other early states had similar statistics. Yet Bachhuber found the greatest impact of the programs came in their first year. How could that be, when almost no one used them?

Another problem with the theory was that even after they took off, medical marijuana programs covered only a small fraction of the adults in any state, even ones like Colorado. At the same time, overall marijuana use began to soar across the United States in 2006. The increase happened both in states that had medical laws and those didn't. In other words, medical marijuana laws were something of a sideshow. The marketing of marijuana as medicine encouraged use across the country, but the new laws themselves made only a modest difference to use.

Yet another problem with the theory was that marijuana simply wasn't a strong enough painkiller to be effective for most people who truly needed opiates. The studies that showed marijuana's effectiveness as a painkiller usually tested it against placebos rather than other painkillers. Like alcohol, cannabis works as an intoxicant first and a painkiller second. And even the modest improvements that cannabis shows may decrease over time. In July 2018, Australian researchers published a study of 1,514 people with chronic pain and found that long-term cannabis use was associated with greater pain over time, and "no evidence that cannabis use reduced prescribed opioid use or increased rates of opioid discontinuation."

A simple look at a map makes obvious that geography more than anything else drove the first stages of the opioid epidemic. From the mid-1990s through 2005, painkiller prescriptions and overdoses spread from Appalachia through the Midwest, with a jump to Florida, which had loose prescribing laws. Addicts and reporters called Oxy-Contin "hillbilly heroin."

The medical marijuana wave was also geographically driven, but on the other side of the country. Until 2008, fewer than a dozen states had legalized medical marijuana. They were nearly all west of the Mississippi. That geographic coincidence — and nothing else — is the most likely explanation for the link that the *JAMA Internal Medicine* paper found.

After 2010, the medical marijuana movement moved east, and the opiate epidemic spread nationally. Suddenly many states had both severe opiate problems and medical marijuana laws. If medical marijuana really offered a solution to the overdose crisis, the evidence after 2010 should have been incredibly strong.

But it isn't. In fact, the post-2010 data shows that medical marijuana laws are correlated with an increase in prescription deaths. Increase, not decrease.

How can I be so sure?

Because I've run the numbers.

Or, to be more accurate, Sandy Gordon has. Dr. Sanford Gordon is a professor at New York University and an expert in data analysis. He's also an old friend. Running correlations on a multiyear dataset with thousands of data points was beyond me, but I knew he would have no problem with it. By his standards, the question I had was simple: Do medical marijuana laws, and changes in state use rates more generally, increase or decrease opiate overdose deaths? And what about cocaine, marijuana's friend from the 1970s?

Finding state-level data on marijuana use, cocaine use, and overdose death rates is easy enough. The Centers for Disease Control tracks overdose deaths. A federal agency called the Substance Abuse and Mental Health Services Administration tracks drug, alcohol, and tobacco use at the state and national level. All the data is public and available for free.

We spent a sunny spring morning downloading it. Then Gordon plugged it into an analysis program called Stata and created a statistical model to run the numbers. Once Gordon had set up the model, we didn't have to wait long for the answer.

As I looked at the numbers I had a sense of how Sven Andréasson or Mary Cannon must have felt when they found a cannabis-psychosis link: people need to see this.

From 1999 through 2016, the most recent

year for which state-level data was available, no link between medical marijuana laws and opiate deaths existed. In other words, the effect in Bachhuber's paper disappeared after 2010.

Further, on a state-by-state basis, overall marijuana use showed a moderately positive link with overall opiate deaths. In other words, states where more people used cannabis tended to have more overdoses.

The analysis also revealed a connection between marijuana and cocaine. Cocaine use fell during most of the aughts and bottomed around 2010. Since then it has risen nationally along with marijuana use — especially among young adults. On a state-level basis the results are even more striking. Marijuana use is strongly correlated with cocaine use at the state level, and changes in marijuana use are correlated with changes in cocaine use.

Other studies since the *JAMA* paper have also suggested that trying to use cannabis to stem the opiate epidemic is a dangerous mistake. A February 2018 paper in the *International Journal of Drug Policy* that studied 245 poor women in San Francisco showed that those who used marijuana were more than twice as likely to use opioids as those who didn't. No other factors — not even homelessness or exposure to violence — increased opiate use nearly as much.

And a July 2017 paper in the *Journal of Opioid Management* found that medical cannabis laws were associated with a 22 percent increase in age-adjusted opioid-related mortality between 2011 and 2014. Worse, mortality increased as time passed.

"It was surprising for me too, when I ran the numbers and got the results," said Elyse Phillips, the study's author. "When you just look at yes or no having a medical marijuana law, there was a correlation with those states having much higher deaths."

But practically no one has noticed Phillips's paper. It has been cited only once in the year since it was published.

An even more worrisome result came from a 2017 study that traced drug use in individuals over time rather than depending on state-level data. Trying to tease out all the factors driving marijuana or opiate use in an entire state is next to impossible. Looking at changes in individual behavior over a period of years is a far better way to determine cause and effect.

So what scientists really needed was a big national survey that asked people about their drug use and then returned to the same people years later. But no one seemed to have conducted that research.

Then Dr. Mark Olfson, a psychiatrist at Columbia University who specializes in addiction, realized that he could find the data in a survey initially designed to measure alcohol use. In 2001–2002 and again three years later, the National Institute on Alcohol Abuse and Alcoholism surveyed 34,000 Americans on their substance use and psychiatric problems.

The study was called the National Epidemiologic Survey on Alcohol and Related Conditions. It focused on alcohol — but it covered other drugs, too. It also had plenty of questions on other risk factors, those tricky confounders.

Olfson and his coauthors examined whether people who used cannabis but not opiates in 2001 were more likely than people who didn't use cannabis to start using opiates over the next three years. The answer was yes. Cannabis users were almost three times as likely to be using opiates in 2004, even after adjusting for other potential risks. The risk was even greater for people who used cannabis heavily. Those people had a 4 percent chance of becoming addicted to opiates three years later, while other people had a 0.5 percent chance — a risk of 1 in 25 versus 1 in 200.

Olfson and his coauthors published their study in the January 2018 issue of the *American Journal of Psychiatry.* "Adults who use cannabis, three years later, controlling for a wide range of things, were found to be at greater risk of opioid use and opioid use disorders," Olfson told me.

Yet Olfson's paper has gone practically unnoticed. In the first eight months after it was posted online, it was cited by other scientific researchers only six times and received little media attention. Olfson says the lack of interest puzzles him. Brain studies of cannabis and real-world experience offer evidence that marijuana use might lead to use of other drugs, he said.

"Initial experiences with marijuana are often pleasurable, they may encourage continued use, they may encourage use of other drugs," he said. "There's evidence that there's a shared underlying biology."

I asked Bachhuber if he would talk about his *JAMA Internal Medicine* paper. He readily agreed. He seemed like a nice guy, genuinely concerned about the welfare of his patients. He's a specialist in internal medicine — an old-school front-line doctor. He said he decided to study the issue after hearing from patients who had used cannabis for their pain.

"I just became really interested in the idea that medical cannabis has been emerging as a treatment option," he said. "What might this increased access to cannabis have on opioid-related issues?"

Bachhuber said he wasn't a strong advocate for marijuana at the time he carried out his study, though he leaned toward legalization. "I had a general liberal attitude about it, but also tempered by medical training, which is extremely negative about cannabis." He was pleased with his findings and doubly pleased the study had received so much attention.

I asked Bachhuber about the fact that the later data doesn't support his pre-2010 findings. He didn't disagree, but he said that finding didn't change the truth of his paper. "When you're looking at the effect of a policy, it may have different impacts over different periods of time."

The updated results have not changed his point of view on medical cannabis, he said. In fact, he believes more strongly than ever that cannabis should be legal. He treats patients who are trying to use cannabis to wean themselves from opioids, sometimes with success. "The story that people substitute cannabis for prescription opioids is really common," he said. "I've never seen it harm anyone yet."

I've never seen it harm anyone yet. The language struck me. It was so similar to the insistence that marijuana has never killed anyone, despite the death certificates that tell a different story. Of course, marijuana is safer than fentanyl. Hang gliding without a glider is probably safer than fentanyl.

But never?

Never is an advocate's word.

Bachhuber has every right to advocate for cannabis legalization, and not to go out of his way to discuss the more recent findings. But his study, which is deeply flawed, has been taken as gospel. That misimpression is not his fault. It's the fault of everyone who is looking for a quick and easy solution to the opiate crisis.

In 2017, Dr. Chinazo Cunningham, one of Bachhuber's colleagues, criticized a federal commission that had noted the findings from Mark Olfson's study showing that cannabis users were much more likely to become opioid addicts.

"People are dying every day from opioid overdoses," Cunningham told CNN. "We must act now."

Do something! Act now! But sometimes doing something is worse than doing nothing. The same urge to do something —

anything — about patients' pain fueled the opiate mess.

A few days before I spoke to Bachhuber, I talked to Dr. Michael Lynskey. Lynskey was the lead author on the Australian and Dutch twin studies that showed that teenagers who used cannabis were more likely to use other drugs later. He's a professor of addiction at — inevitably — the Institute of Psychiatry. I asked him what he thought of the theory that medical cannabis can somehow substitute for opiates.

Lynskey chose his words carefully. "It's something that I think everyone really hopes is true," he said.

But Lynskey came back to a point that other researchers had made. Studies that try to tease out effects by looking at large groups of people provide far weaker evidence than research examining how individuals change over time. And even tracking individuals doesn't always work. For example, observational studies show that older people who exercise are less likely to get dementia. But when researchers tested exercise in a clinical trial of 500 older people with mild dementia, they found that the group that exercised wound up with more symptoms by the end of the trial.

The reason scientists view clinical trials as

the gold standard of research is that those trials take two groups of people who otherwise are almost exactly alike and give one group a drug that the other doesn't get. If the groups are different afterward, it is reasonable to assume that the drug is responsible.

But anything less than a randomized trial is guesswork, to a greater or lesser degree. And ecological studies like Bachhuber's are barely better than nothing. In a February 2018 editorial in the journal *Addiction,* leading experts on drug use called the evidence for the cannabis-stops-opiate use hypothesis "very weak."

Lynskey has spent his career studying addiction. But unlike Bachhuber, he is careful about making any claims about cannabis, positive or negative. Lynskey even cautioned against reading too much into the twin studies, his own work.

"I'm not a clinician — I've got a PhD, and I mainly do statistics," he said. "With my training, we tend to be cautious." He said he understood the pressure that physicians like Bachhuber felt. "Doctors are presented every day with people who are in pain and need relief . . . people will become advocates for something based on their personal experience."

Lynskey tries very hard to avoid becoming an advocate. Drug use and addiction are complex, he said. Being wrong means pushing for policies that can lead to more addiction, more ruined lives.

"My approach, and I've been criticized for it, is to try not to be a particularly strong advocate for anything, because a lot of my work is trying to delve into uncertainty."

So, is the gateway effect true? Does cannabis use make people more likely to use harder drugs? I asked. Lynskey didn't exactly say yes, but he didn't say no, either.

"There's been a number of studies that have used different ways to address this question and have been unable to disprove this association." The social effects of cannabis use might be more responsible than brain changes the drug causes, he said. People who use drugs tend to spend time with other drug users, and if one person in a group tries opiates or cocaine, the others may follow.

As with groups of friends, so with entire nations. What's gone unnoticed in the discussion over state-by-state changes is the striking correlation between the opiate epidemic and cannabis use at the national level. The United States and Canada are outliers among Western countries for marijuana use. Adult and young adult marijuana use have risen sharply since 2005. Meanwhile, Britain has gone the other way.

In many other ways, the United States, Britain, and Canada have a lot in common. They are all wealthy, English-speaking countries with sophisticated health care systems and a long history of opiate use.

While the United States and Canada are suffering an epidemic of overdose deaths, Britain isn't. In 2000, the United Kingdom and the United States had similar drug death rates. That year, about 17,000 Americans and 3,000 people in England and Wales died of overdoses — a death rate of about 6 people per 100,000. On both sides of the Atlantic, about half of those died from opiates.

In 2016, about 65,000 Americans died from overdoses, including almost 45,000 from opiates. In England and Wales, the number was 3,700, including 2,000 opiate deaths. Americans now die from drugs at three times the rate of people in the United Kingdom. And the overdose epidemic in Canada is nearly as bad as that in the United States.

Richard Friedman was more right than he knew in his *New York Times* piece:

If cannabis were actually a dangerous gateway drug, as the attorney general suggested, it would be very easy to see in the data. We would find that medical-marijuana laws increased opiate drug use and overdose deaths.

So they have.

Of course, drawing conclusions based on national-level changes is even more dangerous than drawing them based on changes by state. Many factors — including prescription painkiller advertising, the rise of fentanyl, and possibly even increased Medicaid access — have driven the American opiate epidemic. Attributing all of it to rising cannabis use is clearly wrong. Opiate deaths began rising in the late 1990s, years before American and Canadian marijuana use spiked.

But if marijuana use prevents opioid use, why are overdose deaths centered in the two industrial countries with the highest rates of cannabis use?

Why have they doubled in the decade since marijuana use took off in the United States and Canada?

I don't expect cannabis advocates to have a convincing answer to that question anytime soon.

EIGHT:
STUDY AFTER STUDY
AFTER STUDY

As journalists spread the feel-good myth about cannabis as a cure for opiates, hard evidence linking the drug to psychosis kept coming, from all over the world:

- "Association Between Cannabis Use and Psychosis-Related Outcomes Using Sibling Pair Analysis in a Cohort of Young Adults," *Archives of General Psychiatry*, May 2010: 3,801 participants in Australia: Using cannabis beginning at age 15 raised risk of hallucinations by almost 3 times at 21.
- "Linking Substance Use with Symptoms of Subclinical Psychosis in a Community Cohort over 30 Years," *Addiction*, 2011: 591 participants in Switzerland: Using cannabis regularly in adolescence raised risk of paranoid ideas such as "Someone else can control my thoughts" by 2.6 times.

213

- "Substance-induced Psychoses Converting into Schizophrenia: A Register-based Study of 18,478 Finnish Inpatient Cases, *Journal of Clinical Psychiatry,* January 2013: Almost half of patients hospitalized with cannabis psychosis were diagnosed with schizophrenia within eight years. Psychosis caused by other drugs had lower rates of conversion, with alcohol at 5 percent.

- "Association of Combined Patterns of Tobacco and Cannabis Use in Adolescence with Psychotic Experiences," *JAMA Psychiatry,* January 2018: 5,300 participants in England: Teenage cannabis use roughly tripled the risk of psychotic symptoms; tobacco use did not show a risk after adjusting for cannabis use.

- "Adolescent Cannabis Use, Baseline Prodromal Syndromes, and the Risk of Psychosis," *British Journal of Psychiatry,* March 2018: 6,534 participants in Finland: Using cannabis more than five times raised the risk of psychotic disorders almost sevenfold; after adjusting for parental psychosis and other variables, cannabis tripled the risk.

In all, the studies covered tens of thousands of people in a half-dozen countries, though not the United States, as if American researchers didn't think the issue worthy of their attention.

Along the way, genetic studies progressed enough to enable scientists to rule out one possible explanation for the link. Skeptics had questioned if cannabis use and psychosis were both evidence of an underlying genetic disorder.

Researchers created a database of people who had schizophrenia and examined their genes to see how they differed from healthy people. The scientists found dozens of different genes carried small risks for the disease. But when they looked at whether people with those genes were more likely to smoke marijuana, researchers found a small effect — which extended past cannabis to other drugs, too. In other words, the genes linked to schizophrenia did not cause marijuana smoking, though they may generally contribute to risky behaviors such as drug use.

The reverse was also true. Cannabis raised the risk of schizophrenia both in people who already had higher than usual genetic odds of developing the disease, such as the siblings of people with schizophrenia, and those at normal risk.

In other words, THC was a risk indepen-dent of genetic factors.

Two final pieces of evidence on THC's dangers came from unlikely sources: drug companies looking for weight-loss medicines and drug users trying to get high in a way toxicology screens wouldn't detect.

In the 1990s, pharmaceutical companies began studying ways to turn off the CB1 receptor. The companies knew that mari-juana could increase appetite by activating the receptor. They hoped turning it off would do the opposite. By the early 2000s, they had found chemicals called "inverse agonists," which could lock the receptor in an off position. In studies, the drugs caused significant weight loss.

In 2006, European drug regulators al-lowed Sanofi-Aventis, a French pharmaceu-tical company, to start selling an inverse agonist called rimonabant in Europe. The Food and Drug Administration wasn't as sure. People taking rimonabant for a year lost 11 pounds more than those taking a placebo. But clinical trials revealed the drug caused anxiety, depression, and suicidal thinking. In animal trials, it had caused seizures. In 2007, the FDA recommended against approval.

A year later, with reports of psychiatric side effects mounting, the European regulators reversed course and told Sanofi to stop selling rimonabant. The company suspended sales in November 2008. Other drug makers soon mothballed similar programs, realizing the problem wasn't specific to rimonabant but was an unavoidable problem with the way the drugs affected the brain — what scientists call a class effect.

But THC activated the CB1 receptor, while rimonabant shut it off. So maybe the psychiatric problems rimonabant caused didn't mean anything for THC.

Yet even as problems with rimonabant became clear, users began to suffer severe side effects from another group of manmade chemicals — and these activated the receptor. Called synthetic cannabinoids, the drugs worked similarly to THC and produced a marijuana-like high. The synthetic cannabinoids hadn't undergone years of human clinical trials like rimonabant. They were made by chemists in clandestine labs and sold in corner stores rather than dispensed at pharmacies.

But they too offered real-world proof of the dangers of meddling with the endocannabinoid system.

Design and development of the synthetics

began after the discovery of the CB1 receptor in 1988. At a conference in Ottawa, Canada, a Harvard-trained chemist named John Huffman heard that the National Institute on Drug Abuse wanted ways to test the receptor. Huffman became interested in the research, and especially in finding chemicals that would activate the receptor more powerfully than THC.

Now in his mid-eighties, Huffman is prickly and often declines interview requests. But in 2018, with his beloved Chicago Cubs playing an afternoon game in the background, he agreed to talk about his work.

"It turned out that these were compounds that structurally were very different from THC," he said. "Most people think of the receptor as a lock and key, but that's not right. Receptors are proteins, and they can change shape."

Huffman synthesized many different chemicals that activated the CB1 receptor — and named them for himself: JWH-018, JWH-073, et cetera. Huffman designed his "synthetic cannabinoids" to lock to the receptor more powerfully than THC. Think of the difference between morphine and fentanyl. Morphine occurs naturally. Fentanyl is a synthetic chemical that activates the brain's opioid receptors more strongly, and so fentanyl produces a stronger high and has a much greater overdose risk.

By 1993, Huffman began publishing research on the new chemicals. He had tested them in animals, not humans, so he couldn't be sure they had psychoactive effects. There's no way to ask a mouse if it's high. But Huffman and his collaborators assumed the synthetics would mimic THC's effects on the brain.

"We assumed that if they bound to the CB1 receptor they would be psychoactive." Huffman says he didn't care. As far as he was concerned, the chemicals weren't intended for human use. In 1997, Huffman and his collaborators published a paper describing JWH-018 in detail.

"JWH-018 turned out to be very potent and easy to make," he said.

It was legal, too. Chemists soon realized its potential as a recreational drug. They produced it and other synthetics and sprayed them on herbs. Distributors then marketed them in packets under brand names like K2. The packets included disingenuous labels calling them incense not meant for human use, but word of them spread quickly among smokers looking for a cheap high. The drugs were readily available, cheap, and for a while invisible on toxicology screens.

Unfortunately, they also had severe side effects. People who had no history of psychosis could develop it after using the synthetics a handful of times — or even once.

Truly terrible case reports followed.

An orthopedic surgeon in Louisiana reported on a graduate student "found with his hands aflame on his kitchen stove" after he smoked a synthetic cannabinoid called Black Diamond. The patient, who had no history of psychiatric illness and claimed never to have used any synthetics before, lost most of his right arm and his left hand.

In 2015, a South Carolina man named Timothy Ray Jones allegedly strangled four of his children and beat the fifth to death while under the influence of the synthetics, then put their bodies in his car and drove around with them for days. According to an arrest warrant, he told police that he'd killed the children — aged 8, 7, 6, 2, and 1 — out of self-defense.

"They turn out to be quite toxic in humans, cause all kinds of nasty effects psychologically," Huffman said. He added that he felt no responsibility for the misuse of the drugs. In fact, he was annoyed anyone would blame him. "One is responsible for one's own actions, and if the actions are stupid you have only yourself to blame."

Despite their obvious dangers, restricting the drugs took years. Scientists can't simply be barred from creating a new chemical, or people arrested for possessing it, until drug enforcement agencies have determined it is unsafe. And each different chemical is supposed to be restricted on its own, although agencies sometimes try to restrict several closely related compounds at once. But synthetic cannabinoids were difficult to restrict that way, because many distinct chemical structures could activate the CB1 receptor. The Drug Enforcement Administration banned JWH-018 and four other synthetics in February 2011. By then underground chemists had found other chemicals with the same effects. Even now the DEA and its European counterparts are stuck playing what amounts to whack-a-mole with the manufacturers of synthetic cannabinoids as well as synthetic opioids.

The only good news is that synthetic cannabinoids cause such unpleasant side effects that their use seems to have peaked around 2015 and dropped since. Like LSD and PCP, they are niche drugs. Most people don't want to risk full-on psychosis even if the reward is euphoria.

Marijuana's advocates went to great lengths to explain that synthetic cannabinoids were not cannabis. Cannabis was natural, a plant, not a man-made chemical. But in states that have legalized cannabis, many people no longer use the plant at all. They prefer pure THC, dosed to the milligram. They make no pretense of wanting anything but the high that THC creates when it lights up their CB1 receptors.

The psychosis-inducing effects of synthetics offered one last, crucial piece of evidence about the risks of cannabis. And so, in January 2017, the National Academy of Medicine examined the thirty years of research that had begun with Sven Andréasson's paper and declared the issue settled.

"The association between cannabis use and development of a psychotic disorder is supported by data synthesized in several good-quality systematic reviews," the NAM wrote. "The magnitude of this association is moderate to large and appears to be dose-dependent . . . The primary literature reviewed by the committee confirms the conclusions of the systematic reviews."

But almost no one noticed the National Academy report. The *New York Times* published an online summary of its findings —

in May 2018, more than a year after it appeared. It has not changed the public policy debate around marijuana in the United States or perceptions of the safety of the drug.

After more than a year of working on this book, sometimes I felt like the only people who understood the link between marijuana and psychosis were the scientists who'd studied it, the psychiatrists who'd treated it — and the people who'd seen it for themselves or their family members.

NINE:
STORIES FROM THE
FRONT LINES

Drugs never scared Eric.

Eric came of age in the 1970s in a well-to-do family in New Jersey. Drugs were in the air, and everywhere else. Eric did his share. (Note: Eric spoke on the record about his and his family's experiences. But because one of his sons is a minor, I have used only his first name and changed the first names of his sons. No other details have been changed.)

He saw heroin destroy friends and was mostly priced out of cocaine. "Cocaine was so expensive it was ridiculous." LSD, amphetamines, and especially marijuana were his drugs of choice.

Then Eric married a woman who liked cannabis even more than he did. "She smoked a lot," he told me, his voice gravelly and rough.

No shock, the marriage didn't last. Eric's in his early sixties now, remarried, an artist, designer, and yoga instructor. He'd invited me to his house in upstate New York to tell me his family's story. We sat across from each other at his kitchen table as he talked. The air outside was brisk, but a crackling fire warmed the cozy room around us.

It seemed an unlikely place to discuss marijuana and schizophrenia. But Eric wanted to tell me what had happened to his son, Charles. His candor made him unusual. I'd come across plenty of people who'd had family members become mentally ill after years of smoking. Getting them to talk on the record was difficult. Many parents don't want to admit to themselves, much less the world, that they could have been stricter about marijuana use by their teenage children. At one point I spoke to a physician whose son developed schizophrenia a decade or so ago after years of heavy smoking. He made sure to emphasize that the science hadn't been so convincing back then. I didn't argue the point.

But Eric had reason to talk. He had two sons — Charles, from his first marriage, and Andrew, from his second. Now Andrew was a teenager, and smoking heavily, too. Eric hoped by telling Charles's story to the world he could convince his younger son to stop.

Eric split from Charles's mother when

Charles was in his early teens. The divorce was ugly, and the police called more than once. After living with his mom in New Jersey, Charles moved to Eric's apartment in Manhattan and attended a private school. All along he smoked marijuana practically every day. As his teens progressed he became more defiant. His high school expelled him early his senior year.

"I thought he was just rebellious and difficult," Eric said. "And one day he comes to me and he says, 'I — I'm about to have — I'm really clear that a revelation is coming to me, the revelation of Jesus.' " Eric assumed his son was joking. No, Charles said, he was serious. "I said, 'That may be fine, but we're going to go see a psychiatrist today.' He was seventeen, about to be eighteen." (Charles declined to comment.)

Now Charles was in his early thirties. He had more negative than positive symptoms, Eric said. He heard voices, but he seemed not to have delusions or hallucinations. By the standards of schizophrenia, his disease was relatively mild. Still, it had taken over his life. He'd dropped out of college and worked only in spurts. He survived on government disability checks, which his father supplemented. He'd lived on the streets for short stretches and at one point become so emaciated that Eric worried he would starve.

Into his adolescence, Charles had been handsome, smart, a talented artist and athlete. "He was a great lacrosse player," Eric said. "All that fell apart."

For years, Charles had been unhappy and unpleasant to other people. He knew his life hadn't gone well, but he didn't seem able to change his behavior. He didn't like psychiatrists and refused to take medicine, whether antipsychotics or antidepressants. Eric said he had asked Charles why he wouldn't take medication. "I've gotten used to the music, and I don't want to shut it off, and the drugs shut it off," Charles told him.

After more than a decade of hoping his son would turn his life around, Eric had nearly given up. "He's thirty-two. I'm a realist as opposed to an optimist. I used to think that this is the year he's going to get better, take his medication," he said. "That always leads to disappointment. I've decided to be a realist and hope that he will be incrementally better and find a way forward." (Indeed, Eric emailed me recently to say Charles had found a girlfriend and seemed to be feeling better.)

But Eric faced a fresh worry. He'd remarried and had two more children in his forties. Now Andrew, his son from his second marriage, was using marijuana. Andrew was only 16. He had picked up the habit from older kids at his private high school.

Making matters worse, Andrew's mother — Eric's second wife — had a family history of mental illness, including an uncle with schizophrenia. Eric was not an expert on the statistics that linked cannabis and psychosis. But after seeing what had happened to Charles, he was sure he didn't want Andrew to smoke, especially as a teenager.

Unfortunately, Andrew had ignored his parents's pleas. "He was pretty adamant, 'I'm gonna smoke,'" Eric said. "He just didn't think it was a problem, everybody does it, what's the big deal."

In an interview, Andrew confirmed his father's account. He'd begun smoking along with friends as a ninth-grader. By midway through sophomore year he was smoking or vaping every day. Marijuana is more popular with him and his friends because it is much easier to buy and use than alcohol, he said. It doesn't cause hangovers. "You take a couple hits and then you're having a good time and then it wears off."

At first, Eric and his wife had tried to limit rather than ban Andrew's use. They'd given him a written contract: he couldn't keep marijuana or drug paraphernalia in his room and could use only "occasionally" — once or twice a month. "The ink wasn't dry on that contract before he started breaking it," Eric said. "We'd find him stoned in the morning — he'd get up in the morning and smoke dope." Eric grew even more worried at Andrew's rationale. "He said, 'It makes me feel better,' " Eric said. "I said, 'Why do you need to feel better, what's wrong?' "

He and his wife are moving Andrew to a different school, hoping he would find new friends who smoked less. Andrew is still using, though more recently he has cut back. "He's agreed to be drug-tested," Eric said. "He says he's going to stop for a month." Eric wasn't sure he and his wife could convince Andrew to stop completely, but they had to try — and hope in the meantime his use didn't have long-term consequences. "We're gonna keep on this," he said.

Now a junior, Andrew said he was not happy about having to switch schools. He doesn't believe he has a problem with the drug. He's spoken to his brother about it. "He says you know you have a problem when getting high isn't fun any more."

On the other side of the United States, David Louis Bragen wanted to share his own story about marijuana and psychosis. Bragen grew up in Southern California and moved to the Bay Area with his family in the late 1970s. Marijuana was as popular in Northern California then as it is now, and Bragen became a heavy smoker. At 17, he broke down.

"Reality became different, I came to not be able to tell the difference between commonplace reality and pictures and the visions in my mind and the voices that I was hearing," he said. "Something was definitely going wrong, and I could feel it very deeply." His father brought him to a hospital. It was 1980.

"The doctor that first diagnosed me with schizophrenia told me that if I continued to smoke marijuana, I'm going to continue to end up in hospitals," Bragen said. "And it turned out to be true."

Bragen kept smoking — and relapsing. "One of the things that really got to me was the paranoia, and when I smoked the pot the paranoia got worse, and I had to go to the hospital." He would fixate on the idea that someone in another city was talking to him and making fun of him, and he couldn't answer because the person was so far away.

For twenty years, Bragen's life stagnated.

He tried to major in music at college but couldn't finish. He joined several failed bands. Yet he found giving up marijuana difficult. Many of his friends used the drug. Quitting meant leaving them behind. And he craved the high. "There's something dangerous about it," he said.

During the late 1990s, he slowly cut back. In 1999, he smoked once more — and wound up in the hospital a week later. He decided he would never use again. "I was really ready to call it quits."

Since then, Bragen hasn't used marijuana, and he hasn't been hospitalized. Now he lives in Concord, California, about twenty miles northeast of San Francisco. He survives on disability payments and attends Clubhouse International, a place for people with mental illness to perform structured volunteer work. When we spoke, he sounded satisfied with the direction his life had taken. "My mind is strong enough that I can respond to therapy," he said. "I can keep myself from using."

But Bragen's level of self-awareness is unusual among smokers with psychosis. Many continue to smoke despite repeated hospitalizations.

A Canadian graduate student told me how

he had been diagnosed first with schizo-phreniform syndrome — the milder form of the disease — with a secondary diagnosis of cannabis use disorder, the term psychiatrists use to describe addiction. Now, he has been diagnosed with full-blown schizophrenia.

Still, he continues to smoke.

The student didn't ask for anonymity, but I'll refer to him only by his first initial, A, to protect him. A is the youngest child of a successful immigrant family that moved from the Middle East to Canada. He began smoking at 14 and became a daily user. "Why did I start? I've always been drawn to the forbidden, the illegal," he told me over email. "It was something the cool kids did and my friends. It gave me a huge social community."

A's family has no history of mental ill-ness. His siblings and parents did not know about his cannabis use and wouldn't have approved if they had, he said. He smoked heavily through college but graduated and found a job.

But in his early twenties he felt increas-ingly paranoid. "I quit one job and then another . . . I thought I was being seduced by a woman so that she could charge me with sexual assault, the next job I got through my brother, and I believed he purposely gave me this job to set me up to fail."

He tried again to quit cannabis but didn't feel better. Then he went back to smoking and broke: "I had an episode where I for some reason stopped being able to sleep and went six days [with] no sleep," he said. "Then I drove two hours to visit a friend to tell him about my plan to assassinate Trump, but I didn't trust him, so I changed my mind and drove home. I then attempted suicide." He was hospitalized, discharged, and then readmitted for three months. "I was diagnosed with schizophrenia because I used to believe the news was about me and thought the TV was sending messages."

As of early 2018, A was attending graduate school and looking for work after graduation. But despite advice from his doctors, he still uses. "My smoking is ritualistic. My close friends smoke. We all like to smoke together. I enjoy the high. I now use it while on antipsychotics, so I get zero paranoia or negative side effects."

For now.

Psychiatrists told me they saw stories like A's over and over. Mentally ill cannabis users rarely stop smoking, even after repeated hospitalizations.

"The population that I've treated was a very, very ill population," said Dr. Aneta Lotakov Prince, who worked for several years at a public clinic in Los Angeles County. "There was a group of them that really didn't use anything except for cannabis." Patients quit the drug and improved, she said. Then they started again. "Within a week or two of smoking, the degree of psychotic symptoms that would return was just spectacular."

Prince and other psychiatrists and therapists at the clinic tried to discourage patients from using. Mostly they failed. "It's everywhere, and they get it everywhere — I mean, people deliver this stuff to their doors," she said. "It almost seemed like the more psychotic patients gravitated more to it." The time sequence made the link between cannabis and psychosis obvious to Prince. "Maybe they would stop for a year, two years, and you would think they were in the clear, and then they would relapse."

Of course, many users who have bad experiences with marijuana quit before becoming ill. They're the ones who say, "Weed makes me weird," or "I got paranoid the last time I had an edible, I'm done with it."

But quitting isn't as easy as it seems. First

and foremost, marijuana is addictive. Unlike alcohol or opioids, which produce withdrawal symptoms, cannabis doesn't cause physical addiction. But many users often suffer insomnia, depression, anxiety, and nausea when they try to quit. On surveys, they say they keep using even after the drug causes problems for them, a classic definition of addiction.

About 10 percent of people who have ever tried cannabis become addicted, studies show. That figure understates the true risk, because many people who smoke marijuana do so only once and never use it again. Among people who have tried cannabis more than once, 15 percent or more become addicted, a figure similar to alcohol.

Beyond addiction, many people with psychosis are only vaguely aware they are ill, especially when their symptoms worsen. In the lingo of psychiatry, they lack insight. They don't want to take medicine, and they crave the high that cannabis produces, even if they wind up in the hospital afterward.

And a few people like their delusions, at least at first. They enjoy feeling important, of knowing they are secretly rock stars or being trailed by the CIA. A doctor in Boston told me of a young man whose psychosis took the form of receiving coded messages from his ex-girlfriend telling him that she wanted to be with him. He preferred that delusion to the painful reality of his breakup.

Dr. Melanie Rylander, a psychiatrist in Colorado and assistant professor at the University of Colorado–Denver, said that heavy smokers have extraordinary denial about the drug's impact. "In eleven years of practicing psychiatry, I have yet to convince anyone that marijuana is causing problems for them," she said. "A lot of time those conversations are not very productive."

People with severe mental illness are often so impaired that they lack basic awareness that they are ill, Rylander said. But even people who know something is wrong with their minds rarely connect their symptoms to marijuana. Unlike alcohol, cocaine, or opiates, marijuana rarely causes acute physical crises, she said. Users can tell themselves that their psychiatric problems would have happened anyway.

Dr. Scott Simpson works alongside Rylander in the psychiatric emergency room at Denver Health Medical Center. He said he typically tries to talk around the issue instead of discussing the drug's dangers directly. "Usually my approach is, 'Marijuana is great for you, tell me how things are going for you in general,' " he said.

" 'Why is it that you can't work, why is it that you can't complete school?' "

I could imagine that style working for Simpson. He was friendly and boyish-looking despite the flecks of gray in his hair. Rylander was tall, intense, and angular, but equally thoughtful. Rylander, Simpson, and I were talking in a conference room down a short hallway from Denver Health's psychiatric ER, which came complete with seclusion rooms where seriously psychotic patients could be restrained to their beds.

Simpson told me of a typical case: a man in his early twenties brought in by his parents. "An immigrant family, they are taking care of him . . . he's a pretty sick guy, talks to himself. And, by the way, he smokes pot three times a week."

Marijuana can be "very insidious," he said. Smokers don't think of themselves as addicts. But quitting or even cutting back is difficult. Meanwhile, their psychiatric symptoms worsen little by little. "They have anxiety, new symptoms, and they're smoking pot every day, and it's much more difficult to tease out."

I couldn't help thinking of what George Francis William Ewens had written in the *Indian Medical Gazette* almost 114 years before:

There is, however, equally little doubt that any form of the drug produces a violent craving for it, that the amount taken is gradually increased, and that apart from the physical effect a general moral deterioration, as in alcoholism, sooner or latter [*sic*] sets in . . .

As I talked to Rylander and Simpson, tens of thousands of people gathered a mile to the north for Denver's annual Mile High 420 Festival. It was April 20, the unofficial cannabis holiday. Billed as the largest cannabis-themed event that day anywhere in the world, the festival was a free concert at Denver's Civic Center Park, with Lil Wayne as the headliner. On my way to the hospital, I had walked through lines of people waiting to pass through security screening.

The crowds were a mix of white, brown, and black, mostly teenagers and twenty-somethings. Some were committed smokers who had traveled to Colorado for the festival. On my flight to Denver days before, one of my seatmates told me he'd come to check it out. Dozens of police cars lined the eastern edge of the festival grounds, and LED signs warned that smoking in public was illegal. But no one seemed particularly worried about being arrested. Vendors sold brightly colored bowls and T-shirts.

Nearby, cannabis dispensaries were packed. Would-be buyers milled in the lobbies, waiting for their names to be called so they could enter locked storerooms and choose from dozens of strains of marijuana and THC concentrate.

Within a few hours, some of those users would arrive at Denver Health. As Simpson told me later, in the dry language of medicine, the hospital's medical and psychiatric emergency rooms had "several cannabis-related presentations" that day.

But as Rylander, Simpson, and I spoke, the ward around us was still quiet. Should psychiatrists speak out about what they were seeing to discourage cannabis use, I asked? Simpson said that in Colorado, psychiatrists had tried and failed. "We've put it out there, and the community is not receptive." At this point, his job as a physician was to try to deal with the wreckage, "treat what comes in the door."

What did he think would happen in five years, I asked? What would the Denver Health emergency room be like, especially if cannabis continued to grow in popularity?

Simpson had a three-word answer: "It'll be busier."

TEN:
AN EPIDEMIC ARRIVES

It'll be busier.

Those words cut to the heart of the last defense put up by doubters of the link between cannabis and mental illness. As other evidence has piled up, they've offered it more and more.

If cannabis causes psychosis, why haven't psychosis rates risen in countries along with cannabis use?

At first glance, the rebuttal seems persuasive.

It isn't.

Scientists and health agencies track disease rates in two ways. They count the number of people who have received a new diagnosis in a given period — usually a year — as well as the overall number who have the illness. The first figure is called the *incidence* of the disease. The second is its *prevalence*.

For mental illness in general, and schizophrenia in particular, the United States can't count either number. The federal government doesn't track incidence by requiring that doctors report new diagnoses of serious mental illness to a central database. It doesn't track prevalence through a national registry counting patients. In fact, in November 2017, the National Institute of Mental Health suddenly cut its estimates for the prevalence of schizophrenia in the United States from 1.1 percent of adults to 0.3 percent.

The new figure implied that instead of having almost 3 million adults with schizophrenia, the United States instead had fewer than 1 million. The agency quietly put the new, lower estimate on its website without asking for comment — until Dr. E. Fuller Torrey, a longtime schizophrenia researcher, wrote a scathing opinion piece about the change in *Psychiatric Times.* "Although he has been the director of the National Institute of Mental Health (NIMH) for less than two years, Dr. Joshua Gordon has made 2 million individuals with schizophrenia disappear," Torrey wrote. "NIMH has not said where they went but officially, they no longer exist. This is a remarkable accomplishment."

Torrey pointed out that the new estimate was based on a survey more than 15 years old that specifically excluded people in hospitals, prisons, or on the street — all places where many people with schizophrenia live. Northern European nations make serious efforts to count cases, Torrey wrote. "Compared with these countries, the data available in the US on the prevalence of schizophrenia are equivalent to the data available in some developing countries."

In his response, the NIMH director admitted that the United States didn't know how many Americans had schizophrenia. The institute had "settled on" the 0.3 percent estimate because it believed the old figure was too high. But it wasn't sure the lower figure "necessarily reflects the full picture" either, he wrote. In fact, the institute has now once again updated its website. It now uses a range — from 0.25 percent to 0.64 percent.

Even if the United States did a better job counting cases, psychiatrists agree schizophrenia is a problematic diagnosis. It covers symptoms, not causes. It is a little like diagnosing a patient as "crawling" without knowing if he's on the ground because of a broken leg or a stroke. It overlaps with bipolar disorder, with psychosis, depressive psychosis, schizoaffective disorder, and schizophreniform syndrome. All are treated with antipsychotic drugs.

The common thread in these illnesses is psychosis. But counting psychosis cases is even harder than tracking people with schizophrenia, especially without a national registry. A patient might be diagnosed with bipolar disorder, rediagnosed as having schizophrenia, then called schizophreniform a few years later. That's one patient counted three times.

Making matters even trickier, some big studies show that schizophrenia fell modestly in industrialized countries from 1960 to 1990. No one is sure why, or even if the decrease was real. Some researchers think better prenatal nutrition and obstetric care led to a genuine decline. Others say that as psychiatric hospitals closed, and patients returned to the community for treatment, doctors became more reluctant to stigmatize them as schizophrenic.

"With respect to psychosis incidence overall, there's no good evidence that rates are changing," said Dr. James Kirkbride, an epidemiologist at University College London who led a 2012 study that examined schizophrenia rates in England between 1950 and 2009. Schizophrenia diagnoses dropped, but other psychosis diagnoses rose. More recently, rates of drug-induced psychosis have risen, but from a low baseline, Kirkbride said.

But everyone agrees that the growth in marijuana use from the late 1960s through about 1980 couldn't have done much to psychosis rates. Most cannabis then simply didn't contain enough THC to matter except to very frequent users. Those people may have been at extra risk. But they accounted for a tiny fraction of the overall population — not enough to affect overall rates of mental illness.

But beginning in the 1990s, cannabis became far more potent. The number of smokers rose too. Since 2000, the United States and Canada have seen further increases, while use has risen in some European countries and been flat or down in others. But potency has continued to increase everywhere.

Marijuana users generally start smoking between 14 and 19; first-time psychotic breaks most often occur from 19 to 24 for men, 21 to 27 for women. In other words, almost no one develops a permanent psychotic illness the first time he uses marijuana — or even after a few months. The gap between when people start smoking and when they break averages six years, according to a 2016 paper in the *Australian & New*

Zealand Journal of Psychiatry that examined previous research. The Finnish paper showing that almost half of cannabis psychosis diagnoses convert to schizophrenia within eight years is more evidence of the time lag. A problem that seems temporary becomes permanent.

The time lag is crucial. It implies that the 1990s increase in cannabis use — and the increase in potency that began then and continues today — wouldn't have immediately affected psychosis rates. Instead, if marijuana slowly drives some people into permanent psychosis, rates of schizophrenia and other psychotic disorders might have trended higher in the 2000s, with the increase visible after 2010.

That trend is exactly what some research has found.

Not surprisingly, the strongest evidence comes from northern Europe, where countries can track mental illness more precisely.

The first red flag came from one of the world's most remote areas. In 2016, Finnish researchers reported that rates of psychotic disorders had nearly doubled between 1993 and 2013 in people born in Oulu and Lapland provinces, the country's two northernmost regions.

The study began more than fifty years ago.

First, scientists tracked everyone born in the area in 1966, more than twelve thousand babies. Twenty years later, scientists began another study, tracking every infant born in the area in 1986.

When they compared the generations, the researchers found that the people born in 1966 had a 1 percent chance of being diagnosed with schizophrenia or other psychoses by age 27. The people born in 1986 had a 1.9 percent chance of a psychotic disorder by age 27 — a near-doubling of the risk.

The researchers said they did not know what had driven the increase, though they noted it might be due to improvements in Finland's mental health care system. They published their findings in the journal *Epidemiology and Psychiatric Sciences* in March 2016. The paper received little attention.

By American standards, Finland is relatively drug-free. But the rise in psychosis followed a sharp increase in cannabis use there. Surveys show that use doubled among Finnish teens and young adults between 1992 and 2002 and remained at the higher levels through 2010.

A separate 2009 study of schizophrenia across Finland found a similar trend. New admissions rose from the early 1990s through 2006. The fraction of admissions that included a diagnosis of drug abuse rose from 1 percent to almost 10 percent after 2000. (Cannabis use was not broken out separately from other drugs, but the use of drugs like cocaine is very rare in Finland.)

In other words, marijuana use, psychosis diagnoses generally, and psychosis diagnoses that were specifically drug-related all rose side by side in Finland.

On the other side of the Baltic Sea, a similarly troubling trend took place. Researchers in Denmark recently examined that country's mental illness registry to see if the incidence of schizophrenia had changed between 2000 and 2012.

They found a striking increase. Schizophrenia diagnoses rose about 30 percent. The Danish researchers published their findings in the journal *Schizophrenia Research* in October 2016. Like their Finnish counterparts, the Danish researchers couldn't pin down a reason for the increase in schizophrenia.

But like Finland, Denmark saw a big increase in cannabis use during the 1990s. A 1994 government survey showed that fewer than 4 percent of people aged 16 to 24 had used the drug in the last month. By 2000, the rate doubled to 8 percent. It stayed there through 2010.

In other words, the Danish experience exactly paralleled what happened in Finland.

So, what about the United States?

Again, the short answer is no one knows. Considering that the agency that oversees mental health research here can't even decide whether 1 million or 3 million Americans have schizophrenia, marijuana would have to cause a massive increase in psychosis before anyone would notice.

And unlike Europe, the United States has had two separate waves of growth in marijuana use — first in the 1990s, then more recently, since 2006. The more recent period is particularly striking because adults, not teens, have had the biggest increases in cannabis consumption. Among adolescents 12 to 17, use has risen only in the last couple of years. In fact, dangerous behavior generally has fallen in teens since 2000, although the trend may now be starting to reverse. (Researchers are not sure why. One theory is that tobacco is the ultimate gateway drug, and the sharp decline in teen cigarette smoking has decreased all kinds of risky behavior — though the more recent rise in vaping may be undoing that progress.)

Put all those facts together, along with the time lag, and even if adolescent cannabis use sharply raises the risk of psychosis, proof of a population-wide increase across the United States won't exist for years.

But some evidence has already surfaced. Researchers for Kaiser Permanente and another health insurer recently looked at rates of newly diagnosed psychosis among patients from 2007 through 2012. The insurers cover almost 5 million people aged 15 to 59, the age group the researchers studied. And they are in areas with heavy cannabis use — Colorado, the Pacific Northwest, and California.

The researchers examined electronic medical records across hospitals, mental health clinics, and doctors' offices. They then double-checked a sample of the diagnoses to make sure they were accurate. They specifically excluded cases of dementia-related psychosis, which becomes more common after 50.

Using this more comprehensive approach, they found psychosis rates higher than many previous reports. In their study, which was published in May 2017 in the journal *Psychiatric Services,* they reported that 86 out of 100,000 people aged 15 to 29 received a new diagnosis of schizophrenia, bipolar disorder with psychosis, or other psychosis each year. Based on that figure, the average person has about a 1.3 percent risk of being diagnosed with a psychotic disorder before age 30.

An even bigger surprise came when they looked at adults from age 30 to 59. Psychiatrists expect schizophrenia and bipolar disorder to become obvious by the late twenties. But the researchers found that 46 out of 100,000 people in the over-30 group received a new psychosis diagnosis every year. "The high proportion of true cases in this sample presenting after age 30 contrasts with conventional wisdom that first onset of psychosis typically occurs at younger ages," Dr. Gregory Simon, the study's lead author, wrote.

Translated nationally, the researchers' findings suggested that 115,000 Americans aged 15 to 59 will develop a psychotic disorder every year, Simon wrote. Almost 3 percent of people will receive a psychotic diagnosis before age 60 — 1 person in 35. And that figure probably underestimates the true prevalence, because adults who are uninsured, covered by Medicaid, or in prison are much more likely to have psychosis than those functioning well enough to have private insurance like Kaiser.

(Kirkbride, the British epidemiologist, says the most comprehensive studies show that 4 percent is a reasonable figure for the prevalence of adult psychosis, though only a minority of those people will be diagnosed with schizophrenia.)

Of course, that estimate doesn't mean all those adults are actively psychotic at any time. Some people recover completely. Others get by with antipsychotics. Still others die relatively young — an ugly but real reason that the overall prevalence of people with psychosis can't be determined just by adding up new cases every year.

Still, the Kaiser study suggests that psychosis is a quiet epidemic. If its figures are accurate, Americans under 50 are nearly half as likely to be diagnosed with psychotic disorders as cancer.

The paper did not directly examine whether marijuana had led to any psychotic diagnoses. But it hints at a cannabis-psychosis link in a couple of ways.

First, the fact that new cases are high in marijuana-friendly states may only be coincidence, or a result of the comprehensive counting techniques the researchers used. But it might also be evidence that cannabis was causing more mental illness in Colorado and other high-use states as early as 2007.

Another hint might be if the number of cases trended higher over the six-year period. (Unfortunately, Dr. Simon turned down an interview request, and the paper doesn't break out data by year.)

The second effect is more speculative. Even cannabis advocates acknowledge the drug can speed the development of schizophrenia. But they argue those people would have been psychotic anyway. The cases are accelerated, not caused, they say.

But if marijuana causes psychosis in otherwise healthy people, its neurotoxic effects might not be limited to teenagers and young adults. In other words, marijuana may cause schizophrenia to develop more quickly in young people who are already on the precipice — but it may also slowly cause psychosis in adults who are outside the usual window for the disorder.

That result is precisely what the *Psychiatric Services* paper found. Many adults over 30 are becoming newly psychotic every year.

What is causing all those breaks?

Dr. Erik Messamore believes marijuana is a big part of the answer, and he has a theory as to exactly why prolonged exposure to THC might be neurotoxic.

Messamore, a psychiatrist in Ohio, runs a clinic specializing in schizophrenia treatment. He focuses on helping patients having their first break, or "first-episode psychosis." Evidence shows that the more quickly people are treated, the more quickly they recover. "If you can get people into remission from psychosis within a year, they have much better outcomes," he said.

Messamore began his career with a PhD in pharmacology, intending to research drug development. But he decided he wanted to help people more directly and went to medical school. He is relatively optimistic about his profession. Antipsychotics don't work for everyone, and their side effects are real, but they help for many patients, he says. "Half or more of people with schizophrenia by the modern definition will have meaningful recovery," he said — though the disease may still impair their lives.

After completing his residency in psychiatry at the Oregon Health & Science University in Portland, Messamore worked at an outpatient clinic there, treating patients who had common mental health issues like depression or insomnia.

Along the way he noticed an odd trend.

Messamore's patients were often in their thirties and forties, with no history of psychosis. Many used cannabis. "Oregon is an exceptionally green state," he said. A patient would fail to show for an appointment, then another — and Messamore would learn he had been hospitalized with a psychotic break.

"There'd be no hint whatsoever of any abnormalities," he said. Psychiatrists learn to look for subtle signs of psychosis that other people don't notice: jumbled speech patterns, emotional flatness. Messamore's outpatients didn't have those, much less more obvious problems such as delusions or hallucinations.

Until, suddenly, they did.

The experience wasn't common, but it happened enough to make an impression. Messamore was also working at a state psychiatric hospital, where he saw devastating cases of schizophrenia, patients whom even the strongest antipsychotics couldn't help. They too had something in common. "I had this hard, solid core of patients for whom almost nothing worked," he said. "And among this group they'd almost all been heavy [marijuana] users from their early teens."

In 2013, Messamore moved to Ohio to practice at the Sibcy House, a high-end private psychiatric medical center associated with the University of Cincinnati. The Sibcy patients generally had private insurance. They weren't poor. They had families, jobs, and sometimes advanced degrees. They also had severe psychosis.

A surprising number of them seemed to have used only cannabis and no other drugs before their breaks. The disease they'd developed looked like schizophrenia, but it had developed later — and their prognosis seemed to be worse. Their delusions and paranoia hardly responded to antipsychotics.

How often had he seen these cases, I asked?

"Once a month."

After about two years, Messamore left Sibcy to become an associate professor at Northeast Ohio Medical University and run his clinic. But he is convinced that long-term marijuana use can cause mental illness. He has developed a theory as to how cannabis exposure might harm the brain.

Anandamide, the natural cannabinoid that triggers the CB1 receptor, is known to play a role in the brain's inflammatory processes. Inflammation is a normal response when the body is repairing damage or fighting infection. But prolonged inflammation damages everything from blood vessels to nerve cells. In the brain, chronic inflammation is connected with dementia and other degeneration.

Messamore points to studies showing that long-term marijuana use may be associated with an increase in the enzymes that break down anandamide. That part of the theory is biologically plausible. THC turns on the CB1 receptor, overwhelming the cannabinoid system. The brain has no way to know that THC and not anandamide has caused the extra activity. It might try to bring itself back to normal by reducing its anandamide levels.

But ultimately, that response could cause a shortage of anandamide — thus leaving the brain open to long-term inflammation and increasing the risk of psychosis.

Messamore's theory is unproven and could be wrong. But other psychiatrists I asked said it was worthy of further study. Messamore notes that his theory suggests that patients whose schizophrenia is caused by cannabis may have more inflammation in their brains than those with other types of schizophrenia. Inflammation leaves specific markers, so neuroscientists may be able to test that part of the theory.

Even if his theory is wrong, Messamore believes researchers will eventually discover a biological mechanism that links cannabis and psychosis. He is disappointed that other psychiatrists have not spoken more aggressively about marijuana's dangers.

"They're very, very slow to act in the public interest," he said. "This is something that is an extremely important public health problem, and it is going to be of disastrous consequence to a number of people."

It is going to be, and it already is.

It'll be busier, Scott Simpson had told me about his Denver Health psychiatric ER.

He was only half-right. It — along with its cousins all over the country — is busier already. And marijuana is part of the reason.

The number of people arriving at emergency rooms with marijuana-related problems has soared in the last decade. In 2014, the most recent year for which full data is available, emergency rooms saw more than 1.1 million cases that included a diagnosis of marijuana abuse or dependence — up from fewer than 400,000 in 2006.

Cases involving marijuana rose far faster than those involving cocaine — and even faster than those involving opiates. In 2006, cannabis cases were less common than the other two drugs. By 2014, they were more common than opiates and twice as common as cocaine. Only alcohol, which is far more widely used, contributed to more emergency visits.

Those figures come from a giant government database called HCUP, the Healthcare Cost and Utilization Project. The federal Agency for Healthcare Research and Quality manages HCUP, which uses billing records to track emergency room visits and inpatient hospital stays. Emergency rooms now receive about 140 million patients a year — though that figure doesn't mean 140 million different Americans are going every year, since some people wind up in the emergency room over and over.

HCUP created the emergency room database in 2006. It uses billing records to track more than one-fifth of ER trips nationally. In 2014, it covered 31 million visits to 950 emergency rooms in 34 states — enough to paint a nationally representative picture. The database contains information about everything from the procedures patients undergo to whether they are admitted, discharged, or die. It includes all the diagnoses that patients are given, not just the main one.

HCUP makes limited data, like case counts for different diagnoses, available for free on its website at www.hcup-us.ahrq.gov/. When I found the database, the trends in the free data immediately struck me.

Besides the huge increase in marijuana use disorder, the database showed a big rise in psychosis-related cases. In 2006, emergency rooms saw 553,000 people with a primary diagnosis of schizophrenia, bipolar disorder with psychosis, or other psychosis. By 2014, that number had risen almost 50 percent, to 810,000. Including cases where psychosis was either a primary or secondary diagnosis, the increase was even faster, from 1.26 million in 2006 to almost 2.1 million in 2014.

I wanted to be sure the increase was real, since the American health care system puts a premium on "upcoding." That word is a fancy name for not-quite-insurance fraud — making the most severe diagnosis possible to maximize insurance reimbursements. But upcoding long predates 2006. And the Agency for Healthcare Research and Quality, which has its own psychiatric epidemiologist on staff, told me that it doesn't believe that upcoding or diagnostic changes caused the increase.

For whatever reason, lots more people are showing up at emergency rooms with psychosis — and with marijuana addiction.

But the crucial question was whether the

two problems were occurring together. I needed to count cases where a patient had a primary diagnosis of psychosis and a secondary diagnosis of marijuana abuse or dependence. That combination is a proxy for cannabis psychosis, especially in cases where cannabis is the only drug a patient is abusing.

As far as I could tell, no one had conducted that research. I couldn't find it in any journal. Once again, I turned to my friend Sanford Gordon for help.

Gordon was not thrilled, especially once he realized how much work coding his analysis program to grind through these massive datasets would be. But he said he would.

Fortunately, 2006 is a good starting point for the emergency department data, because adult marijuana use in the United States began rising about then. If cannabis does cause a significant amount of psychosis, the change in the overlapping figures should be obvious.

Through the spring of 2018, we wrangled the databases for an answer. Actually, Gordon wrangled. I tried not to get in the way. Finally, on a sunny Friday afternoon in June, Gordon emailed me the answers.

In 2006, about 30,000 emergency room

patients had a primary diagnosis of psychosis and a secondary marijuana use disorder. Eight years later, that number had almost tripled, to nearly 90,000. Put another way, every day in 2014 almost 250 people showed up at emergency rooms all over the United States with psychosis and marijuana dependence. They accounted for more than 10 percent of all the cases of primary psychosis in emergency rooms. Most of those patients had problems only with cannabis, not other drugs, our analysis found.

Those figures understate the problem. Gordon and I used a conservative definition of psychosis, excluding many people with bipolar disorder. If those patients are included, the number is closer to 170,000. And the HCUP data doesn't provide a way to track occasional users. It includes only patients whose marijuana use was so severe that physicians diagnosed them with abuse or dependence. (The HCUP dataset does include a separate diagnosis for "drug-induced psychosis," which also rose rapidly. But it's impossible to know from that diagnostic code whether the drug was marijuana or something else, so I didn't include it.)

Marijuana disorder was also associated with more severe psychosis — as measured by being hospitalized instead of released following emergency treatment. Psychotic patients with a marijuana sub-diagnosis were about twice as likely to wind up hospitalized as those who didn't have one.

Finally, the emergency room data showed that marijuana dependency was linked to opiate and cocaine addiction. The number of emergency room patients who had a primary diagnosis of opiate addiction and a secondary diagnosis of marijuana use disorder nearly tripled between 2006 and 2014 — more evidence that the theory that marijuana can help people stop using opiates is dangerously wrong.

For cocaine, the link was even stronger. In 2014, almost 15 percent of people who had a primary diagnosis of cocaine dependence or abuse also had a marijuana use problem.

Without reviewing charts or interviewing patients, it is impossible to confirm every case. But the trend is sharp and obvious. Marijuana use and potency rose between 2006 and 2014. Marijuana-related emergency room visits — for psychosis or any other reason — rose even faster.

HCUP's inpatient data shows similar trends over a longer period, since the group has collected data on inpatients since 1993.

The number of hospital inpatients has

remained roughly flat at around 35 million for the last 25 years. But the number of those patients with a primary or secondary diagnosis of cannabis abuse has soared. It rose from 96,000 in 1993 to 300,000 in 2006 to more than 600,000 in 2014. Those numbers don't include people treated at psychiatric hospitals or Veterans Administration hospitals.

Seeing that trend led me to ask Gordon if he would run the same screen on the inpatient data as he already had on the emergency room visits. The long pause that followed let me know that I had pretty much used up my favors. But he agreed.

Gordon found that the situation for inpatients was similar to that for emergency room visitors. The number of cases where a patient had a primary psychotic diagnosis and a secondary diagnosis of cannabis abuse rose 70 percent between 2006 and 2014. By then, people who had a cannabis abuse diagnosis accounted for more than 15 percent of all the psychosis cases that American hospitals treated — far more than any other drug. Again, in most of those cases, marijuana was the only drug being abused.

The annual federal survey on drug use and mental health offers more evidence that cannabis is now leading to increases in mental illness significant enough to be seen at the national level.

Every year, the Substance Abuse and Mental Health Services Administration sponsors a survey of drug use and mental illness among 70,000 Americans.

The survey does not try to count different types of disorders, lumping them into one umbrella category of "serious mental illness." So it cannot be used to make estimates of the prevalence of schizophrenia or other psychotic disorders. Still, without a federal registry, the study is the best source of national data on mental illness.

SAMHSA released data from the 2017 survey in September. It found a marked rise in serious mental illness in the United States too, especially among adults 18 to 25, the heaviest users of cannabis.

According to the study, about 2.5 million young adults met the criteria for serious mental illness in 2017, a rise of more than 25 percent from the previous year and *double* the rate in 2008. Suicidal thoughts and suicide attempts — which both depression and psychosis can trigger — soared, too.

And though the survey does not break down psychotic disorders from other forms of serious mental illness, it showed that inpatient treatment among young adults has risen even *more* rapidly. In 2017, 220,000 young adults received inpatient treatment, compared to 178,000 in 2016 and 97,000 in 2008. People with psychotic disorders are much more likely to be hospitalized than those with depression, so that increase is still more evidence that psychosis is increasing among young American adults.

What's especially striking is that adolescents 12 to 17 don't show the same increases in cannabis use, or in severe mental illness.

Further, about *10 percent* of all cannabis-using adults over 18 met the criteria for serious mental illness in 2017, and another 25 percent met the criteria for less severe conditions. In contrast, among nonusing adults, fewer than 4 percent met the criteria for serious mental illness, and 13 percent for other mental illness.

I know I've just given you an all-you-can-eat buffet of numbers. They can all blend together, and I understand if you skimmed that previous section. But I decided to include them because cannabis advocates so often insist that real-world proof that psychosis is increasing doesn't exist. They're wrong. No one goes to an emergency room for a fun Friday night or is admitted to a hospital for a psychotic disorder on a whim.

Considering the relatively short time frame of the data, these are huge increases. More than 1 million times in 2014, Americans were told that their marijuana use was a diagnosable medical problem. Not by loser friends who don't know how to have a good time. Not by cranky parents who just can't chill. By emergency room doctors.

Imagine if marijuana were actually *dangerous.*

The epidemic isn't coming. It's here.

Why hasn't anyone noticed?

In part because cannabis psychosis is the drug equivalent of a car accident, a semiprivate incident that doesn't make news unless someone is injured. People rarely broadcast that they have been hospitalized for psychotic episodes. When celebrities are involved, news sometimes trickles out. Even then the privacy of mental health information means that the story is often murky.

During 2017, the *Saturday Night Live* comedian Pete Davidson disclosed he'd suffered repeated "mental breakdowns" after years of smoking marijuana. Davidson had been a vocal cannabis supporter. In a 2016 interview with *Rolling Stone,* he had called himself a "pothead."

Then, in March 2017, he announced on Instagram that he had entered rehab. He elaborated in a podcast interview in September 2017, explaining that he had gone into treatment after months of quasi-psychotic episodes related to his cannabis use:

Around October, I would say, September, of last year, I started having these mental breakdowns, where I would freak out . . . blind rage . . .

I had no memory of it . . . I wouldn't know what would happen until I broke something or after I came to, so I was under the assumption that maybe it's the weed, you know, I never really did any other drugs . . .

He went on to explain that he could not stay sober after finishing treatment:

I get off weed . . . [and] I got out, and then I started smoking weed again . . . Two months go by, and I just snapped, I was smoking weed every day, I just like snapped, and I had a really bad mental breakdown . . .

Davidson didn't elaborate on his "really bad" episode. But he said he had initially been diagnosed with bipolar disorder and

suffered from anxiety and low-grade paranoia:

[I would] think everybody's mad at me,
everybody hates me, I'm gonna lose my
friends, I'm gonna lose my girlfriend, my
family hates me . . .

Ultimately, Davidson was told he had not
cannabis psychosis or bipolar disorder but
borderline personality disorder. That diagnosis is marked by manipulative behavior
and resistance to treatment, neither of
which seemed to be an issue for Davidson.
On the podcast, he sounded puzzled and
upset by his problems. He was taking medicine and going to therapy, he said. "This
whole year has been a fucking nightmare."
(Through his agent, Davidson declined an
interview request.)

Yet despite his efforts to quit and awareness of the problems marijuana had caused
him, Davidson continued to use. "I smoke a
lot of pot — it's really hard for me to
concentrate," he said at a comedy show in
Atlantic City in June 2018. He told the
crowd that before coming onstage, "I got
very, very high."

At about the same time, he told another
interviewer that marijuana was helping his

anxiety and Crohn's disease — a chronic disorder of the digestive tract. As for his previous concerns? "I found out I had a mental disorder. I thought I had a drug problem. It's a completely different thing."

Similarly, the nexus between Kanye West's mental illness and his marijuana use briefly grabbed attention, in August 2017, when lawyers for West sued insurers over a claim related to concerts West canceled after a psychiatric hospitalization.

In November 2016, West walked offstage during a show in Sacramento after ranting at the crowd for several minutes. (In 2015, West had given a similarly incoherent speech at a music award ceremony, during which he said he had smoked "a little something" beforehand.)

Two days after quitting the Sacramento concert, West was hospitalized for psychiatric evaluation in Los Angeles. He was held for eight days for a "debilitating medical condition" and released under "full-time care and supervision," according to the lawsuit he filed.

The incident led West to end his tour, which his representatives had insured through Lloyd's of London — a group of insurance companies — for $10 million against cancellation. West's lawyers asked Lloyd's to pay the policy. But the insurers said they needed to investigate. In August 2017, West's lawyers sued, alleging the insurers were unfairly blaming his marijuana use for the cancellation.

The insurers countersued. They said they could not comment on the specifics of West's hospitalization out of respect for his privacy. But they noted the policy did not cover canceled dates due to "the possession or use of illegal drugs."

In 2018, the two sides resolved the suits without disclosing terms. West went on to blame opiates for his 2016 breakdown. Then, in May 2018, he disclosed he had been recently diagnosed with bipolar disorder, which he called his "superpower." By then the hospitalization and lawsuits had been written off as just another semicomic episode in West's chaotic celebrity life. ("I hate being bipolar it's awesome," his new album cover proclaimed.) No one seemed to connect his diagnosis to his cannabis use.

So it goes. Marijuana, THC, and wax are smoked, vaped, ingested, dabbed. Hundreds of times a day in the United States — and that's a low estimate based on a conservative reading of the HCUP data — psychosis follows.

A hospitalization here, an emergency room freak-out there, an involuntary commitment here. A diagnosis of schizophrenia here, cannabis psychosis there, bipolar disorder with psychosis here — though in that case psychiatrists will likely play down the "with psychosis" aspect to the patient. Bipolar disorder may be a superpower. Psychosis, not so much.

No one notices. Not with the United States now topping 70,000 overdose deaths a year. Not with marijuana's backers shouting its benefits.

Not even when the blood flows.

■ ■ ■ ■

PART THREE:
THE RED TIDE

■ ■ ■ ■

ELEVEN:
LABORATORY STUDIES, REAL-WORLD FACTS

The link between marijuana and mental illness is controversial.

The link between marijuana and violence isn't. Most people don't even know it exists.

That lack of knowledge contrasts with the popular, and accurate, understanding that alcohol can cause aggression and violence. Anyone who's ever been in a bar knows that alcohol disinhibits drinkers. For generations, researchers have studied the connection between drinking and auto accidents, domestic abuse, assaults, and even murder.

Marijuana is the world's most widely used illicit drug, trailing only alcohol as an intoxicant. But despite the historical awareness of the cannabis-violence link, scientists have spent little time examining the connection. Many users simply laugh it off.

The research gap is puzzling. It has probably happened in part because violence research falls between social science and medicine. It is usually run by epidemiologists and public health experts, not doctors. And psychiatrists know far more than non-physicians about the mental health effects of cannabis.

But the lack of research also reflects the spectrum of psychological effects that marijuana provokes. Some smokers have anxiety and paranoia. Others find themselves hungry, euphoric, and dazed.

When researchers test cannabis's effects on aggression in laboratory settings, they find the latter effect dominates. In laboratories, most people are less hostile after they've smoked, less likely to react to provocations. Those studies have fed the view that cannabis can't cause violence, a theory that marijuana advocates heavily promote.

In the words of one comedian, Katt Williams, "the side effects — hungry, happy, sleepy. That's it."

"The conventional wisdom has been that cannabis doesn't increase violence because people tend to be mellow when they're stoned," said Wayne Hall, an Australian professor at the Centre for Youth Substance Abuse Research at the University of Queensland. Hall has researched drug use and addiction for more than thirty years and advised the World Health Organization on the health effects of cannabis. "It's an issue that has not been studied that much."

In fact, a 2008 paper that analyzed earlier research on drug use and crime included only ten studies between 1981 and 2001 which looked at marijuana's impact. Not one of those specifically focused on violent crime; they mostly looked at offenses such as prostitution and shoplifting.

Yet a surprising number of recent studies have linked marijuana and violence.

Seemingly unnoticed by either academic researchers or the media, the studies have piled up in the last decade. They are usually not focused on cannabis. They are designed to look at other issues, like mental illness among murder defendants in Pittsburgh or bullying in American high schools or even fighting among tourists in Spain. Collectively, they cover tens of thousands of participants and violence that ranges from fighting to firearm use to murder.

Over and over, they have found marijuana use or abuse is strongly associated with violence — more strongly than alcohol, in many cases.

- A 2013 paper in the *Journal of Interpersonal Violence* used data from a federal survey of more than 12,400 American high school students to examine the link between alcohol, marijuana, and aggression. The researchers' initial hypothesis, which they published as part of the paper, was that alcohol increased violence while marijuana reduced it.

Instead, they found that students who had recently used marijuana — but not alcohol — were more than three times as likely to be physically aggressive as those who abstained from both, even after adjusting for race and sex. Those who used alcohol, not marijuana, were 2.7 times as likely. (Those who used both were almost 6 times as likely.)

- A 2016 paper in *Psychological Medicine* examined marijuana use and criminal behavior among 400 boys in London who were followed for more than forty years beginning in 1961; their marijuana use was surveyed when they were 18, 32, and 48. The paper found that marijuana use at all three times was associated with a ninefold increase in violent behavior even after adjusting for other variables.
- A 2013 paper in the *American Journal*

of Psychiatry examined all 278 people charged with homicides, excluding vehicular homicides, in Alleghany County, Pennsylvania, between 2001 and 2005. It found that 90 defendants had been diagnosed with cannabis dependence or abuse, compared to 65 with alcohol dependence or abuse.

- A 2008 paper in the *European Journal of Public Health* surveyed 3,000 vacationers aged 16 to 35 in the Spanish resorts of Ibiza and Majorca to find out what factors predicted fighting. Cannabis use doubled the risk. Surprisingly, alcohol use did not change it, except for visitors who were drunk more than five days a week, who had a 2.5 times risk for fighting.

- A 2017 paper in *Social Psychiatry and Psychiatric Epidemiology* surveyed 2,000 young men in Britain and 4,000 in China to see if different factors led to violence in the two countries. Drug abuse was far more common in Britain and associated with a fivefold increase in violence. The study didn't break out marijuana versus other drugs but noted that "young British men overwhelmingly reported misuse of cannabis."

Alcohol abuse was associated with a threefold increase in violence.

Other studies with similar findings included a 2018 paper on patients entering treatment for substance abuse in Brazil, a 2018 paper on people arrested in Maricopa County, Arizona, a 2017 paper on firearm violence, a 2015 study on veterans with posttraumatic stress disorder, a 2009 paper on emergency room patients in Michigan, a 2004 paper on youth offenders in Pittsburgh, and a 1984 paper on prisoners convicted of homicide in New York State.

Recent papers also show that the link extends to violence in relationships:

- A 2018 study in the journal *Translational Issues in Psychological Science* showed that among 269 men who had been court-ordered to treatment for domestic violence, marijuana use was associated with physical, psychological, and sexual violence, even after accounting for alcohol use.
- A 2017 analysis of 11 previous studies in *Drug and Alcohol Dependence* found that marijuana use was associated with a 45 percent increase in violence during dating by adolescents and young

adults, compared to a 70 percent increase for alcohol use.

- A 2012 paper in the *Journal of Interpersonal Violence* examined data from a federal study of 9,421 American teenagers over a 13-year-period. It found that marijuana use was associated with a near-doubling of the risk of committing domestic violence by age 26, even after accounting for factors such as depression and binge drinking. (The study showed that binge drinking was associated with a 31 percent increase in the risk of being a *victim* of domestic violence but a *reduced* risk of being a perpetrator.) "We found that any use of marijuana during adolescence and young adulthood increases the risk of intimate partner violence," the authors wrote. "Consistent users were at greatest risk of perpetration and victimization."

Other data come from government surveys that examine drug use by prisoners or people who have just been arrested. The most striking data came from a now-discontinued survey by the federal Office of National Drug Control Policy, which for several years ran a project that asked thousands of arrestees to provide urine samples and answer questions about their drug use.

In 2013, the study found that roughly half of arrestees in five big cities screened positive for marijuana — far higher than the rates for other drugs. In Sacramento and Denver, the cities in the survey where medical marijuana was legal at the time, the percentages had trended significantly higher since 2008. About 60 percent of arrestees in Sacramento screened positive.

Unfortunately, the office ended the survey after 2013, so more recent data is not available. But the Australian Institute of Criminology runs a similar survey in that country. In 2013, it found that one-third of detainees had used cannabis less than two days before their arrest; 23 percent said they were dependent on the drug, and almost 9 percent of those attributed their arrest to it (though in some of those cases they had been arrested for possession of it).

The Department of Justice also occasionally surveys prisoners about whether they were using drugs before or during their crimes. Because they rely on self-reported data rather than a urine sample, those surveys probably underreport use. Still, they have similar findings. The most recent study covered the 2007–2009 period and found that 22 percent of prisoners in state prisons reported using marijuana at the time of their crime, up from 15 percent in 1997; 63 percent said they were regular users at the time of the crime, up from 58 percent in 1997. All the surveys, whether in the United States or Australia, and whether of new arrestees or long-term prisoners, showed much higher rates of marijuana use than of other drugs.

Taken together, this work implies that marijuana use may be as large or larger a risk for violence as drinking. At the least, it suggests the laboratory research on marijuana and aggression is flawed. Those studies often exclude people who have a history of psychotic disorders. Researchers cannot ethically expose them to cannabis given the known link between the drug and psychosis. And older studies were conducted with marijuana much lower in THC than the high-potency strains smoked today.

As a result, the laboratory work misses the most devastating kind of violence that marijuana provokes.

Alcohol has predictable effects. It disinhibits drinkers and makes them more aggressive, whatever their baseline. Marijuana doesn't cause aggression in everyone. Many users relax. But some become paranoid, and some of those have full-blown psychotic episodes.

Marijuana causes paranoia and psychosis.

That fact is now beyond dispute. Even scientists who aren't sure if marijuana can cause permanent psychosis agree that it can cause temporary paranoia and psychotic episodes. The risk is so obvious that marijuana dispensaries advertise certain strains as less likely to cause paranoia.

Paranoia and psychosis cause violence.

Overwhelming evidence links psychotic disorders and violence, especially murder. Studies have confirmed the connection, across cultures, nations, races, and eras.

The definitive analysis was published in *PLOS Medicine* in 2009. Led by Seena Fazel, a psychiatrist and epidemiologist at Oxford University, researchers examined twenty earlier studies on people with schizophrenia and other forms of psychosis. They found that people with psychosis were 5 times as likely to commit violent crimes as those without it. They were 19.5 times as likely to commit murder. (Amazingly, a 2010 paper in the *American Journal of Psychiatry* on the deaths of young children in Taiwan found almost exactly the same risk ratio. Kids who had a parent with schizophrenia were 19.4 times as likely to die by homicide as those who did not.)

Full-blown schizophrenia is relatively rare. But because people with schizophrenia are so likely to kill, they make up an appreciable fraction of murderers — 5 to 10 percent in most studies.

A 2007 British government study of all 5,884 people convicted of murder in England and Wales in the previous decade found that 348 of the perpetrators, or 6 percent, had a schizophrenia diagnosis. The rates of convictions of people with schizophrenia increased faster than the overall homicide rate over the period.

A broader analysis in 2009 of eighteen international studies found that people with schizophrenia were responsible for 6.5 percent of homicides — about 1 in every 15. Some more recent studies find even higher rates. A 2011 paper by Australian researchers examined 435 homicide cases and found that 9 percent of the killers had a schizophrenia diagnosis.

When researchers include forms of psychosis other than schizophrenia, they find an even stronger link. Studies by the Justice Department and other researchers show that 15 percent to 20 percent of American prisoners have diagnosable psychotic disorders. (The United States has about 2 million people in prison, so those estimates suggest that up to 400,000 American prisoners have psychosis. The number has soared in the last fifty years, as state mental hospitals have closed. Researchers and treatment advocates agree that many mentally ill people who would once have been housed in hospitals are now in prison.)

Marijuana causes psychosis.

Psychosis causes violence.

The obvious implication is that marijuana causes violence.

Yet the marijuana-psychosis-violence connection is even stronger than the *A*-causes-*B*, *B*-causes-*C*, therefore *A*-causes-*C* explanation suggests.

Here's why.

The studies that demonstrate that psychosis causes violence also show that most of that violence occurs when people with psychosis are using drugs.

In other words, when a patient with schizophrenia stays on antipsychotic medicines and away from recreational drugs, he is only moderately more violent than a healthy person.

But many people with schizophrenia do not stay on their antipsychotics for long. And people with psychosis use and abuse drugs far more than the general population — and when they do, they become far, far more likely to commit violent crimes than healthy people do.

Fazel's meta-analysis in 2009 that found people with psychosis had a fivefold increased risk of violence showed that the risk was tenfold when those people were also substance abusers. (It was about double for those who had psychosis but didn't abuse drugs.)

Advocates for the mentally ill put great emphasis on the fact that people with psychosis aren't overly violent if they don't use drugs. But they rarely acknowledge the flip side of the issue, that people with psychosis are frequently drug abusers — and that as a result their overall risk for violence is very high.

"You don't just have an increased risk of one thing — these things occur in clusters," Fazel told me over a coffee in London's hip Borough Market; he'd come in from Oxford for a conference, and I was on my way to the Institute of Psychiatry and Robin Murray. "You have a set of genes that cluster around the difficult things." The difficult things. Like a tendency to murder. The understatement seemed very British.

And the drug that mentally ill people use

the most is marijuana. Unfortunately, its tendency to cause paranoia and psychosis makes it a terrible choice.

A 2018 paper in the journal *African Health Sciences* examining 520 psychotic patients admitted to a South African psychiatric hospital in 2012 and 2013 found that 49 percent had engaged in violent behavior during their psychotic episodes. Of those, most had used cannabis, sometimes alongside methamphetamine.

The 2007 British government survey of homicides found that almost 60 percent of the 348 offenders with schizophrenia were using drugs when they killed. Cannabis accounted for most cases, with cocaine and amphetamine almost all the rest — not surprising, because stimulants can also cause psychosis. The number of murderers who were both psychotic and drug abusing increased far faster than the overall homicide rate over the study period.

It is worth remembering that — in part, thanks to Robin Murray and the Institute of Psychiatry — cannabis use in Britain peaked between 2000 and 2005. Since then, cannabis use has fallen, and the number of homicides committed by people with schizophrenia has also trended lower, according to a more recent British government report.

Few studies have directly examined the interplay between marijuana, mental illness, and violence in depth. Until last June, the most striking came from the Dunedin research. Written by Louise Arseneault and published in 2000 in the *Archives of General Psychiatry,* it showed that people with marijuana dependence had a fourfold risk for violence, even after adjusting for other variables. (People with alcohol dependence had twice the risk, so the Dunedin study is another that demonstrates marijuana is more correlated with violence than alcohol is.) Patients with schizophrenia or schizophrenia spectrum disorders had 2.5 times the risk of the average person.

But the most stunning figure covered people who had both a cannabis disorder and a schizophrenia spectrum diagnosis. Those people were 18 times as likely to commit violence as the average person. Even that figure may understate the connection between marijuana, mental illness, and murder. Because the Dunedin study was so small, it used broad measures for violence. But Fazel's 2009 paper showed that the more severe the crime, the higher the risk that a psychotic person would commit it.

In other words, in people predisposed to

delusions, marijuana seems to function as a supercharger for sudden, extreme violence. Their underlying fears make them prone to lash out uncontrollably if cannabis provokes their paranoia. In a study published in the *Medical Journal of Australia* in 2006, of 88 murderers with psychosis in Australia, 50 reported delusional beliefs that the victim was threatening them or needed to be killed to save other people; 52 of the killers reported being dependent on marijuana.

In 2013, researchers in Italy examined violence in 1,582 psychiatric patients in Southern Italy and found another strong link. In their paper, which was published in *Rivista di psichiatra — Journal of Psychiatry* — they reported drug users were almost 9 times as likely to become violent as patients who didn't use. Eighty percent of drug users "exhibited violent behavior," and cannabis was the most frequent drug of abuse.

Even after adjusting for age, gender, and type of psychiatric illness, using marijuana caused a roughly four-fold increase in the risk of violence leading to injuries, the researchers reported. "Cannabis use/abuse is associated with violent behavior inflicted on the self and others, and constitutes a specific risk factor." The researchers also noted the unpredictability of violence associated with cannabis. "Violent behavior was correlated only to cannabis use/abuse and had a tendency to recur, being 'immediate' and therefore difficult to predict."

Then, last June, Swiss psychiatrists examined violent behavior among 240 young psychotic patients in their clinics.

Over a three-year period, 62 of the 240 became violent, which researchers defined as "an assault causing any degree of injury, any use of a weapon or any sexual assault." Three patients attempted or committed murder.

In other words, these patients had a 1-in-4 chance of becoming violent over a three-year period — even though they were in treatment, and even though Switzerland has low crime rates overall.

The researchers then looked at the risks for violence. In a 2017 paper in the journal *Early Intervention in Psychiatry,* they examined various potential causes, including substance abuse — though they didn't specifically focus on cannabis. Patients who lacked insight into their psychosis were more violent, they found. But that finding wasn't a huge surprise, and the differences were relatively small.

Then the researchers reanalyzed the data,

this time comparing the 82 patients who were dependent on cannabis with the 158 who were not. Their new paper appeared online in *Frontiers in Psychiatry* on June 14, 2018. It found an extraordinary association between cannabis and violence.

Psychotic patients with a cannabis use disorder had a nearly 50 percent chance of committing violence during the three years of the study. Those who weren't using had only a 15 percent chance. When researchers adjusted for other variables, such as alcohol use or adherence to treatment, the gap increased. The cannabis-dependent patients were four times as likely to be violent. No other factor was nearly as important. Alcohol use, which was common among the patients, made no difference.

I emailed Valerie Moulin, the psychiatrist who led the study, to ask why she had decided to check specifically for the effects of marijuana. "At first I wasn't particularly looking for this link between cannabis and violence," she wrote back. "I was more interested in poly-consumption (alcohol and cannabis, in particular), because we thought it was what was relevant."

But her experiences with patients — along with discussions with other psychiatrists and the handful of recent papers showing the cannabis-violence risk — led her to look again. "We were surprised by this link," she wrote. "Now we need to look at it to try to minimize violence."

Moulin encouraged other researchers looking at violence and psychosis to split out cannabis rather than lumping it with other illicit drugs. "It was a mistake to mix everything up, and it overshadowed the understanding of the effects of cannabis."

But much more work remains to be done, Moulin wrote. She will continue her research to see if she can tease out why cannabis-using patients are so prone to violence — and whether the risk increases over time.

Moulin added that she believes marijuana's tendency to cause violence probably occurs not only in patients with preexisting psychosis but in otherwise healthy people. "The trend is towards a major effect of cannabis use," she wrote.

Harry Anslinger might have been a racist jerk, but eighty-five years ago, he was right about marijuana.

TWELVE:
AXES AND KNIVES

So where are all the heinous murders committed by psychotic cannabis users?

Turns out they are all over, hiding in plain sight.

Scientists like to say that the plural of *anecdote* is not *data.* In other words, don't draw conclusions based on stories, no matter how convincing they sound. Just because you know someone whose toddler was diagnosed with autism a week after a vaccination doesn't mean vaccines cause autism. (They don't.)

But no one ever points out the statement is true in reverse. If the scientific evidence suggests that a phenomenon is common, then that phenomenon should be easy to spot in the real world. The issue of marijuana and violence proved the point. Once I started looking, I found a long parade of cases, each more terrible than the rest.

Are all those murders and assaults making

294

a notable difference to crime rates? Very possibly. The first four states that legalized marijuana for recreational use — Alaska, Colorado, Oregon, and Washington — have seen their rates of murder and aggravated assault increase much faster than the United States' rates as a whole since legalization. The gap has increased every year.

Canada, which also has high and rising rates of cannabis use and in 2018 became the first major Western nation to legalize use, has seen a similar trend. Homicides in Canada rose almost 30 percent between 2014 and 2017.

The violence comes in three baskets.

The first is the most obvious and hardest to dispute: murders and assaults by mentally ill people who were also heavy cannabis users.

A second group of crimes is committed by people who became violent from temporary cannabis psychosis.

The third comes from people who weren't obviously psychotic, but whose crimes occurred alongside marijuana use. In those cases, marijuana may function more like alcohol, as an intoxicant that reduces inhibition. Often, those crimes took place in the context of small-time drug dealing. They also included a disturbing number of crimes against children.

Unfortunately, I had no foolproof way to tease out hard numbers for any of the three categories. Like being drunk, cannabis psychosis is a form of voluntary intoxication, which is not a defense to criminal behavior. Defense attorneys raise the issue infrequently.

Nor do police departments or prosecutors particularly care about marijuana use, especially in cases where a defendant's guilt seems beyond dispute. Police officers, detectives, and prosecutors have crimes to solve and cases to prepare. Unless cannabis or cannabis intoxication is relevant to winning conviction, they may not investigate it.

More broadly, the criminal equivalent of the HCUP database — a national dataset showing drug use or abuse by defendants — doesn't exist. Even in murder cases, police sometimes don't run a toxicology screen on a defendant if they arrest him more than a day after the crime. The screens are expensive and won't prove the perpetrator was using drugs at the time of the offense anyway.

The only way to have a complete count of all the serious violence associated with marijuana would be to look at each individual case, a project far beyond my resources.

Only a large team of researchers could examine all the 17,000 homicides committed in the United States last year. For serious but nonlethal violent crimes, the task would be even harder. In 2017, the United States recorded 810,000 aggravated assaults.

So, the cases that follow are just a tiny and nonrandom sample of the marijuana-linked violence that occurs every day. Be warned, though: they make for horrifying reading.

Advocates for the mentally ill often say the media stigmatizes people with schizophrenia by highlighting crimes they've committed. The truth is the opposite. Reporters and news outlets dislike covering these cases, especially when the victims are family members. The crimes are brutal and ugly but without much mystery. People with severe psychosis rarely make much effort to hide what they've done. Even when they do, they are obvious suspects, and police often arrest them quickly. These are the murders the *New York Post* writes about for a day or two and the elite media ignores as tabloid fodder.

Still, the cases popped up frequently. After a while, I grew to recognize murders that involved psychosis even when it wasn't explicitly mentioned. They were chilling both in their lack of obvious motive and in the degree of violence. Often, they involved bats or knives rather than firearms. They were the cases where parents suffocated infant children, or children clubbed their adult parents, or men stabbed to death women they'd never met before in libraries.

Of course, I couldn't always be sure cannabis played a role. Prosecutors don't usually bother with a marijuana charge when they indict someone for beheading his best friend. But mental illness is no barrier to having a Twitter account or a Facebook page.

Over and over, I found that defendants themselves revealed either their love of marijuana or their psychosis or both.

Take Domenic Micheli. His case briefly received national attention because it was so brutal and unusual. Micheli, a personal trainer in Tennessee, allegedly murdered Joel Paavola, his former boss, with a hatchet in June 2018 — in the gym where they had both worked. Micheli was arrested a few days later in Kentucky. He had filled his Facebook page with long, incoherent posts. A few days before the attack, he called himself "The Sun of God." Three months earlier, he'd posted a photo of cannabis buds and a rambling discussion of his cannabis use:

> the other thing is that, marijuana is something that is fun because it gives you truths
>
> if we adjust things so people didn't feel like escaping it will definitely lose a certain aspect of its appeal even from a mathematical standpoint . . .
>
> ill tell you this though, its not all fun and games. i have a weed called mystery kush from mendocino county
>
> this is not my idea of a good time. it feels like the hard part of a painful relationship in some ways. and you can tell its going to be that type of trouble just from the smell . . .

Less than a week after Micheli was arrested, police in Hamden, Connecticut, arrested Kyle Tucker for allegedly beating his mother Donna to death and burning her body in a backyard fire pit. Tucker — a 34-year-old graduate of Harvard Law School — told police that he had killed his mother because she had tried to poison him repeatedly. God "got into my body and walked me downstairs with my baseball bat and it was very quick and almost even hard to remember," he told detectives, according to news articles about his arraignment.

In the months leading up to the murder, Tucker's tweets were increasingly bizarre and had a strong cannabis tint. He asked the president to appoint him ambassador to Jamaica, so he could help local marijuana farmers. "Jamaica has a climate very well suited for the cost-effective production of high-q weed outdoors," he wrote, in one tweet that could have come out of a cannabis industry conference.

Tucker was also obsessed with Bob Marley and the singer Lana Del Rey. Three months before allegedly killing his mother, he made the eerie threat that "if Lana keeps disrespecting me, i'm gonna burn that bitch with a slow bonfire on live television as I smoke weed and laugh in her inferior face."

(Indeed, corpse mutilation happens weirdly frequently in these cases. Dean Lowe, a British man who called himself "the biggest stoner in the world" on his Facebook page, dismembered his girlfriend Kirby Noden after murdering her in January 2017. He then flushed part of Noden's body down the toilet of their apartment in Cornwall, England, left the rest for trash collectors, and made a necklace from her teeth.

Blake Leibel, a would-be movie producer whose Ukrainian girlfriend Iana Kasian complained to her mother that he smoked "huge amounts" of marijuana, scalped Kasian in their West Hollywood apartment in May 2016. When she was autopsied, Kasian had only a teaspoon of blood in her body, according to the *Hollywood Reporter,* which ran a long article about the case. Kasian and Leibel had a 3-week-old baby at the time of the murder.

Camille Balla, a Florida woman with a history of mental illness, gouged out her mother's eyes with broken glass after killing her in March 2018, according to prosecutors. Balla told an ambulance crew that she had just smoked marijuana; investigators found notes that included "religious-themed written messages" about cleansing the soul.

Sometimes the marijuana connection came not out of social media but from the comments of prosecutors. In May 2018, weeks before Micheli was arrested, a Cleveland judge sentenced William T. Jones Jr. to sixty-three years in prison for the murder of a uniformed Salvation Army volunteer in December 2017. Video shows that Jones walked to up to the man, 21-year-old Jared Plesec, and shot him in the head without warning.

After shooting Plesec, Jones did not immediately try to escape. Instead he went on an incoherent four-minute rant that a passerby captured on video. "Fuck Trump," he yelled. "They're going to kill us all." Then he ran off, tried to carjack two vehicles, and wounded several other people before being arrested. At his sentencing hearing, a prosecutor said that blood samples taken from Jones after his arrest tested positive only for marijuana and no other drugs.

Yet — like most other cases I examined — the Jones verdict ended in a guilty plea and prison. Judicial records would not connect it to either marijuana or mental illness. Toxicology reports are part of police investigative files, and in many states, those effectively remain sealed even after a case is closed. The prisoner and arrestee surveys on drug use are years out of date and don't directly examine the connection between marijuana and violence anyway. The lack of readily available information is the reason that counting marijuana-linked cases is so difficult, and probably why the trend has not yet become obvious on a national level.

Proof of the link was easier to come by in cases where the killers also died — either by suicide or by being shot by police officers. Autopsies that include toxicology reports are standard in those cases. And in many states, including cannabis-rich ones like California and Colorado, autopsy reports are public records.

In November 2017, a month before Jones shot Plesec, a man named Kevin Neal went on a rampage in Tehama County, a rural California community 200 miles north of San Francisco. Neal killed five people and wounded nine others before killing himself.

The crime could have been even more devastating. After killing his wife and three neighbors, Neal drove to a local elementary school just as kids were arriving for the day. But a quick-thinking secretary heard shooting as Neal approached. She ordered a lockdown, and the school's front gate was pulled shut before Neal could drive inside. He fired from outside for several minutes before fleeing. Two students inside were shot and wounded, but none was killed. Neal killed one more person before sheriff's deputies pinned him down ten minutes later. After a final exchange of gunfire Neal shot himself. He died at 8:23 a.m., November 14, 2017.

Neal's rampage attracted little attention. In the United States, the murder of five people barely rates as national news. But after seeing that the Tehama County Sheriff had called Neal "deranged [and] paranoid," I asked the sheriff's office for his autopsy report.

I also called his sister, Sheridan Orr. Family members of perpetrators often won't talk, but Orr was a welcome exception. She spent more than an hour walking me through her brother's history of mental illness and violence, which were intimately connected to marijuana.

Neal, Orr, and their sister grew up in an affluent family in North Carolina. Even as a child, Neal had trouble following rules, but he was smart and funny and "got away with it."

In about 1987, when Neal was 14, he and a group of friends began smoking marijuana. The effect was immediate. "He started to get into more and more trouble," Orr said. Within two years, he'd been arrested for the first time. He went to a rehab clinic but continued to smoke. In 1992, he was arrested again, for possession of marijuana with intent to sell.

By then, Neal had become difficult, Orr said. He lived in the basement of their house, but when people walked above him, he became enraged and shot a BB gun at the floorboards. Their parents fought over his behavior. "Honestly, Kevin was the reason they got divorced," Orr said. (Neal's mother, Anne, declined to comment on the record.)

Neal was never properly diagnosed as either having a psychotic, mood, or personality disorder, Orr said. But he was clearly mentally ill. For the next fifteen years he continued to act out — and to smoke marijuana. In 2006, he was arrested again, this time for assault with a deadly weapon. Again, though, his mother hired a lawyer for him. He was not convicted.

By then Neal showed clear paranoia and psychosis. He claimed his neighbors were sneaking into a house his mother had bought him and defecating inside it. He built a large fence around the house — "the crazy fence era," Orr said.

By 2007, he and his girlfriend, Barbara Glisan, had decided to move to California so Neal could become a marijuana farmer. Tehama County is just east of the famous Emerald Triangle, three northern California counties that are famous for high-potency cannabis cultivation.

Orr had little contact with Neal by this point. Both she and her sister were frightened of him. But Neal remained close to their mother, so Orr knew what was happening in his life. In California, Neal began to grow marijuana in bulk. At one point, Orr's mother told Orr she had paid a $20,000 electric bill for him. (Growing cannabis indoors requires huge amounts of electricity.) Orr said that her mother had told her, "You wouldn't believe how good Kevin is at growing marijuana."

Becoming a marijuana farmer did not solve Neal's problems. He was arrested again in 2013, for a hit-and-run. By 2016, he had moved to a decrepit house in the unincorporated community of Rancho Tehama Reserve. Sheriff's department records show he and his neighbors feuded constantly. Neal became convinced, without evidence, that the neighbors were cooking methamphetamine. To retaliate, he would shoot at random, according to calls neighbors made to the sheriff's department.

In January 2017, Neal was arrested again, this time for stabbing a neighbor. He faced felony charges, including assault with a deadly weapon. Neal's mother pledged her house to bail him out, but he faced the serious risk of jail. As the case moved forward, Neal's paranoia worsened. He fired Leo Barone, the lawyer representing him. "He was making bizarre statements," Barone told the *Los Angeles Times* after the shooting. "I confronted him."

Orr said Neal had told Barbara Glisan — by then his wife — to leave him before the shooting, probably because he knew he was on the verge of snapping. Glisan refused. The couple had nine dogs, and she didn't want to leave them. Ultimately, Neal killed Glisan and the dogs the day before he attacked the school.

Given the path Neal's life took, "this is the logical conclusion," Orr said. She blamed both methamphetamine and cannabis for her brother's decline. But Neal's autopsy report showed only THC and no other drugs or alcohol in his blood.

While Neal was troubled his entire adult life, Matthew Riehl's decline was sharper and shorter. Riehl grew up in Colorado, served in the National Guard in the Iraq War, and in 2010 graduated law school from the University of Wyoming. But in the spring of 2014, while practicing law in rural Wyoming, he began sending bizarre texts to his mother, Susan. When she couldn't reach him, she decided to see firsthand if he was all right.

"He was barricaded in his house," she said. "He had aluminum foil all over the windows. He had tubs of water all over the place. And in the spare bedroom, he had a bunch of baby chicks hatching. It was pretty crazy, but he was happy to see me. I talked him into going to the hospital."

Veterans Administration records show Riehl was held in the psychiatric ward of a VA hospital in Wyoming in April 2014. The episode marked the beginning of his unraveling. He fought with family members, made bizarre posts about his former law school, and claimed police officers were harassing him. His brother told University of Wyoming police officers that Riehl had been diagnosed with bipolar disorder.

In 2016, Riehl gave up his Wyoming law license and moved to Douglas County, Colorado, where he shared an apartment with a roommate and posted odd videos on YouTube. He worked at a Walmart for a while, then quit.

Susan told me that Riehl smoked marijuana frequently in Wyoming. "When we would visit with him, sometimes he would smoke in front of us," she said. (Susan later emailed me that she did not believe marijuana played a role in the case.) Riehl may also have been using methamphetamine. In a YouTube video he posted on December 19, 2017, he mentions a burn on his lip, then giggles and adds the burn did not result from cooking meth.

But in the early morning of December 31, 2017, Riehl had no methamphetamine in his system, only caffeine, small amounts of alcohol, and THC — including one form of the drug that is a product of eating rather than smoking cannabis and is particularly psychoactive. (The amount of alcohol in his blood was about the amount from one drink.) Around 3:00 a.m., Riehl called 911 to complain he'd been the victim of domestic violence. When Douglas County sheriff's deputies arrived at his apartment, they found him agitated. But they concluded no crime had occurred and left.

Two hours later, another 911 call brought them back. Riehl was waiting for them. He barricaded himself in his apartment and screamed, "Go away! Go away!" and "Identify! What's your name!"

Then he started shooting. By the time he had finished, Deputy Zackari Parrish was dead, and six other people, including four law-enforcement officers, were wounded. Deputies fired back, killing Riehl.

Because a law-enforcement officer was killed, the Riehl case attracted attention in Colorado. It was the start of a troubling trend. In the next five weeks, two more Colorado law-enforcement officers were killed in separate incidents and six others wounded. The state had not seen so much violence against police officers in such a short period in at least thirty years.

In each case, marijuana appeared to play a role.

Of course, in most encounters in which police and civilians clash with lethal consequences, it's the civilians who wind up dead. Those killings provide another window into the link between THC and violence.

In 2017, police in Colorado killed 35 civilians, accounting for 3.5 percent of all the police-involved killings in the United States that year — though Colorado has only 1.7 percent of the US population. Colorado has a strong open-records law, so I requested autopsy reports on the people who had been killed from several large counties. I received 18 reports back.

Few documents in the world are starker than autopsy findings. They can't be spun or argued away. They hold the brutal truth of a human being's body at the moment of his death — his diseases, his hidden vices, the way he perished.

The Colorado reports revealed that in every one of the eighteen deaths, the person who was killed had drugs in his system. In three of the eighteen, THC was the only drug. (THC is fat-soluble, and the body can store it in a form that is not psychoactive. But toxicology screens distinguish between psychoactive and nonactive forms of the drug. I counted only screens that show the active forms of THC as being positive.) In eight more cases, THC was found alongside other drugs or alcohol.

Alcohol and methamphetamine both trailed cannabis. They were each found alone in two cases and in combination in six more. Opiates, cocaine, and benzodiazepines were found in only a handful of reports combined.

Hungry, happy, sleepy — and primed for lethal conflict with the police.

THIRTEEN:
ONE BAD TRIP

In cases where cannabis caused temporary psychosis in people who otherwise didn't have a history of mental illness, the violence was generally less graphic. But the crimes were if anything more tragic, because the perpetrators often had no criminal history and the violence seemed inexplicable — sometimes even to them.

Occasionally, they attracted national attention, like the curious case of Joseph Hudek.

On July 6, 2017, Joseph Daniel Hudek IV boarded Delta Airlines flight 129, from Seattle to Beijing. His mother worked for Delta, so he had a pass for seat 1D, in first class. He had flown earlier in the day from his hometown of Tampa. While he waited in Seattle for his connection, he bought several 10-milligram THC edibles, legal in Washington state. He ate at least three before boarding and texted a friend that he hoped to sleep for the twelve-hour flight.

He didn't.

According to a flight attendant, Hudek appeared sober and normal at takeoff. About an hour later, with Delta 129 cruising over the north Pacific, he stood and went into the first-class bathroom.

Two minutes later, he emerged — and shouted, "I want to get out!" as he lunged at the airplane's right front cabin door. Two flight attendants jumped him. He fought them off and succeeded in raising the handle halfway. Other first-class passengers saw the melee and scrambled to stop Hudek.

The brawl intensified, and a flight attendant broke a wine bottle over Hudek's head. But Hudek didn't go down. "Do you know who I am?" he yelled. Finally, passengers held Hudek down long enough for flight attendants to put plastic zip-tie cuffs on him. He continued to struggle as the pilots diverted the plane back to Seattle.

"The violence was incredible," one passenger said afterward. "I was afraid he was going to kill the flight attendant."

Hudek had no criminal history, and no history of psychosis or mental illness, though he had used alcohol and marijuana in college. He had flown almost two hundred times before without incident. His lawyer blamed the edibles for his breakdown. In keeping with other cases, US District Court Judge John Coughenour ruled that Hudek's cannabis use could not be used as a defense for his behavior. (I drew on court documents for this narrative; Hudek's lawyer did not return repeated calls or emails for comment.)

In May 2018, Hudek pled guilty to assault and interfering with a flight-crew member. Coughenour sentenced him to two years in prison. "I'm deeply sorry for everything that's happened," he said at his sentencing hearing. Still, he faced disdain and incredulity.

"Tampa man: Edible Marijuana Made Me Punch Out Flight Attendants," the *Tampa Bay Times* wrote. Inevitably, *High Times* argued that "a deranged, violent outburst caused by cannabis sounds more like a myth straight out of *Reefer Madness* than a real possibility." *The Stranger,* an alternative newspaper in Seattle, sneered that "the idea that he simply got too high was Hudek's first defense" before acknowledging edibles could cause severe reactions and suggesting that reformulating them might help.

Still, Hudek was lucky. He didn't get the cabin door open. He didn't have a weapon.

He didn't kill anyone.

He could have.

On March 25, 2018, in South Hill, Washington, a suburban town about thirty-five miles south of Seattle, two cousins and a friend decided to smoke marijuana that they had strengthened with near-pure THC oil extract. The three men went outside and wrestled for a few minutes before going back inside their house to wash up.

Then the cousins argued. And 27-year-old Robert Reynolds snapped, according to charging documents. He picked up a pistol. He told the third man that his cousin, Samuel Boren, was the devil and had come to the house to hurt them. He raised his pistol to Boren. And he pulled the trigger.

Bleeding badly, Boren begged Reynolds to take him to the hospital. Instead Reynolds shot him again and again, until the pistol was empty. Then he asked his friend to sit and hold his hand until he calmed down. Two hours later, he called 911 to report that he had killed his cousin.

"I know I'm a killer, but I don't feel like a murderer," he explained to the deputies who arrested him, according to news reports. After all, he told them, the devil had tried to possess Boren's body.

The *Seattle Times,* the biggest newspaper in the second-biggest cannabis-legal state, didn't write a single article about the case.

On April 4, 2016, in Centennial, Colorado, Kevin Lee Lyons was engaging in his favorite pastime, smoking marijuana. Married, 46, with three children and no criminal record aside from a warrant related to his failure to appear on a civil matter, Lyons had been a contractor. But he'd stopped working months before. Some neighbors called him foul-mouthed and difficult, and his behavior had worsened in the previous two years. His wife Liz attributed the change to a 2014 car accident, though the incident had been so minor that Lyons hadn't bothered to go to the emergency room until hours later.

Lyons had once had problems with alcohol and cocaine, but for years he had attended Alcoholics Anonymous meetings. He no longer drank or used cocaine. Instead, he spent much of his time smoking marijuana in a shed behind his garage. His cannabis use was becoming an issue in his marriage. By the beginning of April, his behavior had become odd enough that Liz had asked him to sleep in their basement. Still, she told police later that she assumed he was depressed and was not worried he would become violent.

That Monday, Liz decided to let their daughter — who had a sore throat — stay home in the morning and then take her to school around noon. When Liz came back home around 1:00 p.m., Lyons shouted, "Who's there?" and began to rant. Liz told her husband she wanted to take him to the hospital. (The district attorney's office for Colorado's 18th Judicial District, which covers Centennial, provided a redacted investigative file about the case; I drew from it for this narrative. Through his lawyer, Lyons declined to comment; Liz also declined to comment.)

The suggestion infuriated Lyons. He made the sign of the cross and told his wife she was the devil, then disappeared into their basement, where he chanted in a mock–Native American style. When he reappeared, he was holding a .45-caliber pistol. "Get out," he said. "I'm not kidding."

Liz left the house and crossed the street. Her neighbor, Laurie Juergens, was outside, gardening, taking advantage of the unseasonably warm early spring day. Still, Liz wasn't running. She would later tell police that even after she saw the pistol she didn't think her husband would hurt her. They'd been together twenty years, had three children. She thought she knew him.

Lyons walked outside, lifted the pistol, shot Liz in the back. *Pop, pop, pop, pop.* Some people heard four shots, others five or six. The suburban neighborhood was so unused to crime that some witnesses didn't realize what they were hearing. One thought the sound was a nail gun.

Liz lay helplessly on Juergens's lawn. Lyons shot Juergens, too, hitting her in the face. Juergens stumbled into her house and Lyons briefly vanished.

In the calm moments that followed, Kenneth R. Atkinson, Juergens's next-door neighbor, ran to rescue Liz. But as he reached her, Lyons reappeared — and shot him.

Severely wounded, Atkinson retreated behind his Chevy Suburban. He gasped for breath while Lyons shouted incoherently. One witness heard Lyons yell, "The Lord is risen." Another remembered him cursing and saying, "This is Indian country."

Lyons crossed the street. He ignored his wife. He would later tell deputies that he believed he'd killed her. (She was bleeding so badly that when paramedics arrived they first thought she was dead.) Instead, he walked to the Chevy Suburban where Atkinson was trying to hide. Lyons shot Atkinson several more times point blank, including at least once in the head, killing him.

When police officers and Arapahoe County sheriffs' deputies arrived, Kevin fired another fusillade and then surrendered without resistance. Just after being cuffed, he told a police officer, "I live here and it's a nice day. In the Bible it says if you kill seven that you will be rewarded seventy times."

His bizarre behavior continued after the arrest. As he was being booked into jail, he again chanted in a mock–Native American style. In his postarrest interview, he told officers that "his wife is a two-headed snake and he had to kill it."

Yet interspersed with psychotic rants, Lyons showed an equally disconcerting friendliness, as if he had no idea what he'd just done. "I love you," he told a neighbor, as he was led into the back of a cruiser. Then he asked officers who would be picking his children up from school.

Neighbors — and Liz — spent months trying to understand Lyons's crime. Whatever his anger issues, he had never been violent before. Liz told police she did not know he even owned a pistol.

In the investigative file, Lyons's cannabis

use pops up again and again. When deputies entered his shed, they noted a strong odor of marijuana and many empty marijuana containers. His toxicology screen found only THC and no other drugs or alcohol aside from two antihistamines, including one sometimes prescribed as a mild antianxiety drug.

In January 2017, Liz told investigators that Lyons had used marijuana habitually for twenty years. "Ms. Lyons said that Mr. Lyons smoked marijuana all day, like a chain smoker of cigarettes . . . she couldn't tell when Mr. Lyons was high or not."

Yet no one seemed to connect Lyons's slow breakdown to the drug, not even his wife. She blamed Lyons's 2014 car accident for his decline. "Ms. Lyons said that in the last year, Mr. Lyons was more isolated and depressed . . . Mr. Lyons was distant and had not drank alcohol in nine or ten months."

In the months after he was arrested, Lyons was held in the Arapahoe County Jail. His psychosis slowly faded, though it did not entirely disappear. His phone calls were recorded and transcribed, standard practice for inmate calls. In some, he said he was still hearing voices, but in general he appeared far more rational.

Just sixteen days after his arrest, a recorded jail call caught him saying, "I'm very normal, very sane. I know what's wrong, I know what's right. I know I have some very serious charges against me." Later, he said, "Tell my kids that I love them and that I'm truly sorry, it will mean something sometime to them. I will not be here for my whole life, I promise you that."

Lyons was wrong.

On June 20, 2016, Judge Carlos Samour found Lyons competent to stand trial. With his guilt never in question, the only question prosecutors faced was whether to ask for the death penalty. Liz begged prosecutors not to do so, but they weren't sure. Atkinson was a doctor, well liked and well respected in the neighborhood. Lyons had executed him as he was wounded and helpless.

Ultimately, though, prosecutors decided not to ask for death. Instead, Lyons pled guilty to first-degree murder. At his sentencing hearing, Laurie Juergens called him "beyond evil" and said he should receive "the harshest penalty this state allows."

Samour sentenced him to life plus 352 years.

As of summer 2018, he was housed in a prison in Buena Vista, about 120 miles southwest of Denver, a jumping-off point for outdoor adventures like hiking, camping, and whitewater rafting. Lyons will never have a chance for those. Colorado's inmate locator says he will finish serving his sentence on December 31, 9998 — the state's way of saying that only death will free him.

Richard Kirk seemed to have an enviable life when he pulled into a Denver dispensary on April 14, 2014, looking for an edible to relieve his back pain. A father of three sons, he arranged his work schedule so he could drop his kids off at school and pick them up afterward. A Mormon, Kirk didn't use marijuana or drink. He had been employed as a graphic designer at the same company for twelve years. He'd been married for almost sixteen years to Kristine, a beautiful blonde who worked in marketing. He'd been attracted to Kristine as soon as he saw her. He followed her from Dallas to Denver. They married barely a year after they met.

"She was trying to get me hooked on Colorado, but I was already hooked on her," he told me in the spring of 2018. We were sitting in a cinderblock room at the Bent County Correctional Facility in Las Animas, Colorado, a quiet town on the state's rugged eastern plains. A table separated us.

A prison employee sat just outside, watching. Nonetheless, prison officials had allowed me a face-to-face meeting with Kirk even though I wasn't a lawyer or a relative. They'd given us several hours to talk. That courtesy made the visit a privilege, a reflection that Kirk was a well-behaved inmate.

Talking about his wife made Kirk tear up. "This June we would have been married twenty years," he said.

But Kirk's life in 2014 was not as idyllic as it first seemed.

For years, he had been dependent on opioid painkillers. The prescriptions had started for back pain, but after a while he couldn't function without them. He regularly finished prescriptions ahead of schedule and cadged pills from friends. A few months before, he had quit. Now he was using again.

Money was another problem. While he and Kristine made close to $150,000 a year combined, Kirk was a spender. Their debt had piled up. Two years before they had gone to a consumer credit service, but their finances were still strained.

So was their marriage. Around 2008, the Kirks had talked about divorce and gone to counseling. More recently, their fighting had picked up. Kristine had been furious after

Kirk failed to make a reservation for a hotel where they planned to vacation with friends.

Nonetheless, at 6:00 p.m. on April 14, 2014, Richard Kirk was an ordinary American, a suburban dad and husband with no history of violence or mental illness. April 14 was a Monday; he'd gone to work. Afterward, he hung out with his youngest son. He ordered Domino's for dinner. Around six, Kristine came home. "I always loved looking at her pull up," he said. " 'Here she is to save the day.' " They were out of milk, so Kristine sent him to Whole Foods for more.

On the way home, with his back hurting — and in mild opiate withdrawal — Kirk saw a sign for The Health Center, a South Denver dispensary. Recreational marijuana had become legal in Colorado four months before. Kirk had voted against the amendment approving it. He'd voted in 2000 against the original Colorado medical marijuana law too. He didn't think marijuana was medicine. "Marijuana's been smoked for a long time, and it's a drug, and it's recreational."

Kirk made a U-turn and pulled into the dispensary.

Ten minutes later, at 6:40 p.m., he was the proud owner of a piece of Karma Kandy

Orange Ginger, a candy edible with 100 milligrams of THC. "I didn't want to smell like smoke," he said. In his driveway, he ate a chunk. About a third, by his recollection. "All I wanted to do was nibble," he said. "I got home, I sat in the driveway, and I just randomly took a bite."

If Kirk hadn't been so eager to take his mind off his aching back, he might have remembered that marijuana hadn't always agreed with him. Living in Dallas in his twenties, he'd been a smoker. "I have had things that I would call paranoia, yes, from smoking marijuana," he said. "That's a common thing, you smoke pot, you get paranoid, you think someone's watching you." Another warning sign: mental illness ran in Kirk's family. A brother had schizophrenia.

Kirk said he had never felt psychosis or hallucinated during his previous marijuana use. Still, the paranoia played a part in his decision to quit smoking. Once, in 2007, he'd smoked while camping with friends. Suddenly he decided he needed to be alone and drove off without telling anyone. He returned hours later, insisting he was fine.

After eating the candy that April 2014 night, he came inside for dinner.

For a while the drug didn't seem to have

any effect. Kirk went into the bathroom to eat another piece.

And he lost his mind.

He was afraid. Then he was terrified. Then the world seemed to end, reality shattering into pieces that Kirk couldn't reassemble. Kirk didn't want the edible anymore. He wanted it out of his body and mind. He stuck his fingers down his throat to vomit it up, but he was far too late. "I didn't think it was marijuana, I thought maybe someone had given me acid or something."

The next minutes are more than a blur but less than a fully formed memory. Even after four years behind bars to think about the night, Kirk couldn't explain to me what had happened — much less why. He crawled through the window of his son's room onto the back deck of his house. "I thought, 'Man this is nothingness out here,' " he said. "Where are they?' " He went back inside and lay down on the floor. "I thought I was on concrete and people were pounding on me . . . my wife was, like, Richard, 'What are you doing — what are you doing?' "

It is unclear exactly when Kirk's psychotic episode started, but Kirk probably ate the candy around 7:00 p.m., and the psychoactive effects of edibles can take an hour or more to hit. In any case, by 9:30 p.m.,

Kirk's behavior had unnerved Kristine enough that she called 911 for help. She told the dispatcher her husband was hallucinating and talking about the end of the world. He had asked her to shoot him and threatened to shoot her.

The Kirks had a pistol in the house. They'd bought it not long before, for no particularly good reason. They lived in one of Denver's safest neighborhoods. Kirk told me he'd bought it in part to scare off wildlife when they camped in the mountains. Kristine's mother and stepfather, who hate Kirk with an understandable passion, told me he'd bought it because his best friend, Patrick Milligan, had recently bought one. "Anything Pat got, Richard had to have," Kristine's stepfather, Wayne Kohnke, told me.

Milligan agreed. "We got a handgun, and then they got a handgun," he said.

Kristine didn't like the pistol much, but she accepted it. Wayne insisted Kirk keep the gun in a safe and bought him one. It was in the safe that night. So, Kristine was frightened, not terrified, when she called 911 — at least at first. The dispatcher didn't make her call a priority. A police station was barely a mile from the Kirk house, but officers didn't arrive for almost fifteen minutes.

By then, Kristine Kirk was dead.

Her fear worsened during the call. She ordered her sons to hide in the basement and asked police to "please hurry." But the dispatcher never told officers of the emergency.

Then her husband unlocked the gun safe.

Maybe the biggest mystery of the night is how Kirk opened the safe, given his condition. He told me it had a finger-button lock with a simple combination, 1-3-2-4, and he thought he had the muscle memory to remember it. His postarrest interview may provide clues too. Kirk alternates between odd references to Jesus and eternity and an equally unsettling caginess. After about twenty minutes, he tells the detective he wants a lawyer, ending the interview.

Kirk took out the pistol. Kristine saw it. She told the dispatcher that her husband had a gun and she had nowhere to hide. As his 7-year-old son watched, Kirk stalked up to his wife. She screamed. He put the pistol to her head and pulled the trigger, killing her instantly. Then he handed the pistol to his son and told the boy to shoot him. When the police arrived, he surrendered quietly.

Experts on violence like to say its causes are "multifactorial." Only psychopaths kill for no reason, the simple thrill of murder. Even in psychosis perpetrators usually pick their targets. Kirk didn't shoot his sons or himself. He killed his wife.

The shooting was, by definition, domestic violence, but Kirk wasn't a stereotypical abuser, and the murder didn't come out of a fight. Kirk simply snapped — murdering his wife, scarring his children forever, and destroying his own life.

Why? Even now Kirk has no idea.

"They all just think I'm a monster, and I did become one," he said. He pled guilty to second-degree murder and received thirty years in prison. His in-laws think the sentence is far too light. "I would have pulled the switch myself," Wayne said, when I asked about the death penalty.

"No one ever talks about the aftermath," Kristine's mother Marti said. "The aftermath is horrendous." At a time when they expected to be happily retired and traveling, she and Wayne have effectively become parents again. "We've got three kids to put through college, we've got three boys to raise." They have cut off contact between Kirk and his sons.

"They hate him," Wayne said. "They loved their mother dearly, and how would they ever trust anyone after the man that was supposed to protect them killed their mother?"

Wayne and Marti had grown to believe their former son-in-law leaned more toward the willful cruelty of psychopathy than the desperate violence of psychosis. But they too were certain that cannabis was behind the murder. "All he needed was that marijuana — no different than alcohol," Wayne said. "Giving him the courage."

Kirk existed at the center of the Venn diagram of three great American maladies — opiate abuse, financial stress, and easy access to firearms. But he'd lived there for years and never been violent, not until he ate a bite of Kandy Karma Orange Ginger.

Patrick Milligan will never understand why Kirk shot his wife.

The Milligans and the Kirks had known each other for almost twenty years. In the year before Kirk killed Kristine, the two couples and their children spent thirty-one weekends together, Milligan said. The five children from the two families called themselves "the wolfpack" and were nearly inseparable. "We were together constantly." Their only real disagreements came when Milligan felt that Kirk let his kids misbehave in public.

"He's not violent, not at all," Milligan said. "The guy is so nonviolent that he wouldn't even spank his kids when they desperately needed it."

Kirk's love for his sons proved the senselessness of the crime, Milligan told me. "An absolute guarantee that he would never see his kids again — do you think he would do this on purpose?

"I think he's a very good person . . . who did the unthinkable."

Unthinkable. Senseless. Pointless. Those words kept coming up in these cases. But then psychosis is the very definition of senselessness.

No crime is more senseless than the death of a child from abuse or neglect. And marijuana use is linked to child fatalities with extraordinary and disturbing frequency.

In two separate cases in late 2017, young couples allegedly abused their children — a 3-month-old in Nevada, a 20-month-old in Idaho — to the point that the children had seizures — and then blew marijuana smoke at their children in the hopes of calming the seizures. Both children died, and all four parents have been charged with murder.

In August 2018, in Lewisville, Texas, Blair Ness allegedly threw his one-year-old son Ashton down on a concrete courtyard, then stabbed the boy to death as horrified neighbors tried to stop him. Neighbors told police Ness was yelling about Jesus; officers found his apartment reeking of marijuana. Ness's girlfriend told police that when she left for work a few hours before, he had been happily feeding the boy. Ness has been charged with capital murder.

In July 2017, in Wyoming, Michigan, Lovily Johnson left her six-month-old Noah in a car seat for more than a day while she smoked marijuana with friends. By the time she returned, he was dead, his corpse decomposing in its seat. (She was charged with murder. Her first trial ended in a hung jury in September 2018.)

Horror stories aren't data. But hard data about child deaths does exist. Federal law requires states to examine child fatalities that are suspected to be related to abuse or neglect, and to publish at least basic data on what they find. ("Abuse" means actively malign behavior, such as shaking or beating

a baby. "Neglect" falls into several categories, such as an intoxicated parent who has
a car accident that kills an infant who wasn't
properly buckled. Either can be criminally
prosecuted.)

Some states, such as New York, offer little
more than case counts in their public
reports. Others provide much more detail
about the deaths and the risk factors associated with them. For the last few years, Texas
has been among the most forthright. Texas
also has more fatalities than any other state,
accounting for 10 to 15 percent of all child
deaths in the United States, depending on
the year. For the 2017 fiscal year, which
ended August 31, 2017, the Texas Department of Family Services reported 172
confirmed child deaths due to abuse or
neglect.

Buried deep inside the state's "FY2017
Child Fatality and Near Fatality Annual
Report" are statistics on drug use by the
people responsible for those deaths. In at
least 90 of the 172 cases, the state determined that perpetrators were using drugs or
alcohol at the time the children in their care
died. (The number was probably higher,
but in 26 cases authorities couldn't be sure.)

Cannabis was by far the most commonly
used drug. Fifty-six perpetrators were

actively using marijuana at the time of the deaths, compared to 23 using alcohol, 16 using cocaine, and 14 using methamphetamine. (The figures total more than 90, because the perpetrators were using more than one drug in some cases.)

Worse, since Texas first began reporting this data for the 2014 fiscal year, marijuana use has risen sharply as a percentage of cases — while other drugs and alcohol have remained roughly constant.

The number of cases is particularly stunning because Texas is a conservative state with relatively little marijuana use. Federal surveys show that in 2016, about 10 percent of adults in Texas said they had used marijuana in the last year, and 6 percent in the last month — both lower than the national averages.

Based on national statistics, about one-third of those monthly users consume cannabis every day. Put another way, only about 1 out of every 50 Texans is a daily marijuana user. Yet in more than one-third of all the child deaths from abuse or neglect in Texas in 2017, authorities found that the perpetrator was using cannabis at the time of the child's death.

The annual reports don't provide enough detail to determine exactly what role marijuana use played in each child's death. Some may be causally linked, homicides following cannabis-induced psychosis, as the Ashton Ness case appears to be. Others may look more like the Noah Johnson case, where cannabis use occurred alongside fatal neglect or accidents. In some cases, the drug may have played no role in the child's death.

Yet the strength of the association cannot be ignored. Marijuana use was more likely to be linked with the death of children than almost any other factor, including domestic violence or mental illness. Once again, researchers who *weren't* looking for evidence that cannabis was linked to violence found it anyway.

FOURTEEN: MYTHS, SPREADING

Marijuana-caused psychosis is an obvious risk for violence. Yet cannabis is associated with a surprising amount of violence even without overt psychosis. The assaults and homicides around small-time marijuana dealing are the most common example. Those happen every day and rarely attract more than local attention.

Sometimes police or news reports mention the perpetrators were using marijuana at the time of the crime. More often they don't, so knowing for certain is impossible. But even if the reports don't specifically mention use, assuming that people dealing or trying to steal marijuana are often using the drug seems reasonable.

All that can be said for sure is that the crimes occur with extraordinary frequency. (Google "marijuana murder" or "marijuana homicide" for yourself.) They range from simple retail rip-offs gone wrong to complicated and premediated robberies, like the case of Garrett Coughlin. Coughlin, a 24-year-old Colorado man with no criminal history, allegedly shot and killed three people in February 2017 at a house west of Denver where marijuana was being illegally grown.

In keeping with the lack of information around cannabis and violence, law-enforcement agencies often lump crimes around marijuana dealing in the broader category of drug crime. Even that classification can be confusing, since drug-related crimes fall in different groups. They include possession, crimes committed to pay for drugs, and trafficking-related conflict, as well as the violence due to drug effects like psychosis or intoxication.

But a few agencies have recently begun to note the amount of violence specifically related to cannabis dealing.

York County, South Carolina, has about 250,000 people. From 2015 through early 2018, 41 people were arrested for homicide there. Twenty-three of those were involved in drug deals. Of those, 17 cases involved marijuana, and either the seller or the buyer was killed. "The most common way to die by homicide in York County is over drug rip-offs involving pot," Willy Thompson, a prosecutor, told the local newspaper.

In June 2018, Atlanta police chief Erika Shields said that many murders in the city were "tied to marijuana, in this day and age of medical marijuana . . . crimes are being committed for it." Shields's comments were particularly striking because Atlanta's homicide rate is so high — about four times the national average. (An Atlanta newspaper called the *Northside Neighbor* reported Shields's comments, which she made to a Rotary Club. Unfortunately, after initially saying through a spokesperson that she was "interested" in an interview, she later declined to speak or provide department statistics.)

Similarly, the Las Vegas police department noted an "emerging trend" in its 2017 annual report "of drug-related altercations where someone gets robbed or killed over a relatively small amount of drugs or marijuana." The number of murders in Las Vegas soared 80 percent between 2011 and 2017, from 79 to 141, even excluding the 58 people killed in the music festival mass shooting in October 2017.

But marijuana is illegal in South Carolina and legal only for limited medical use in Georgia. It was legalized for recreational use in Nevada only in mid-2017. Crimes around dealing might be expected in those states. What about states like Colorado or Washington, where the drug is fully legal and has been for years? Proponents of legalization have long argued moving marijuana onto a regulated market would reduce violence around black-market dealing.

More broadly, they argue marijuana's apparent association with crime also occurs precisely because the drug is illegal. In other words, some law-abiding people will drink alcohol but won't use marijuana, simply because using it inherently means they are breaking the law.

As a result, the population of users inherently excludes some people who are law-abiding and at low risk for violence. As a result, cannabis use may seem to have a spurious association with violence.

If cannabis advocates are correct and those two theories are true, legalizing shouldn't increase violence. In fact, it will likely decrease it by creating a safer state-regulated market.

Unfortunately, the opposite has happened.

George Brauchler, the district attorney for Colorado's 18th Judicial District, which includes Arapahoe County, told me his jurisdiction has seen 11 murder cases since 2012 related to black-market marijuana sales. "All it [legalization] has done is professionalize the black market," Brauchler said.

Colorado residents can now legally keep up to twelve cannabis plants at their homes. But enforcing the twelve-plant limit is difficult. The easiest place to hide an illegal marijuana grow is alongside a legal grow. Police have basically no way of knowing whether a house has twelve plants or twice that many.

Even twelve plants can easily produce 10 pounds or more of marijuana a year, more than even the heaviest smoker can consume. That excess homegrown marijuana and the high-THC wax and shatter made from it can't enter the state system. Instead, it is often sold illegally, for lower prices than the regulated and taxed products sold at dispensaries. On Craigslist, Colorado sellers offer an ounce of shatter for $350; a gram of shatter at a dispensary usually costs $30 or more, or $840 an ounce — though dispensaries cannot legally sell more than eight grams at once.

The price gap has created a thriving and dangerous black market. Both Colorado residents and out-of-state traffickers take advantage, Darcy Kofol, the chief narcotics prosecutor for the 18th District, told me.

As of mid-2018, she spent three-quarters of her time on black-market cannabis cases, not opioids or other drugs. Those deals often come with violence, sometimes pre-planned by either the dealers or the buyers, sometimes spontaneous.

"We've seen a lot of Craigslist violent crimes," Kofol said.

The issue of oversupply and black-market supply in states that legalize has no solution. Marijuana is simply too easy to grow. In Oregon, which gave grower's licenses to almost anyone who wanted one, state regulators reported almost 1 million pounds of legal marijuana piled in warehouses in early 2018 — four ounces for every adult in the state, and three years of supply based on 2017 sales.

As a result, retail prices in Oregon fell in half in the last two years. Some stores in 2018 offered an ounce of marijuana for as little as $50. But they are still higher than black-market prices. Worse, as prices fall in the legal system, the burden of state taxes and regulations increases compared to the overall revenue that growers and dispensaries make. Some smaller, less efficient growers will simply close up shop. Others may shift — or shift back — to the black market.

In other words, legalizing marijuana

doesn't end the black market in marijuana. It just makes the drug cheaper, on both the legal and illegal markets. Those lower prices increase availability and drive up use.

Crime follows.

Cannabis advocates told voters legalization would lower crime by giving police officers a chance to enforce more important laws. "Legalization Will Reduce Crime, Free Up Police Resources" was the headline of an opinion piece by the former Seattle police chief Norm Stamper on CNBC.com in 2010.

Advocates are still sending that message. In August 2017, Senator Cory Booker, a Democrat from New Jersey, introduced a bill to end federal prohibition of cannabis. In his announcement on Facebook Live, Booker linked legalization to falling crime — specifically violent crime.

"You see what's starting to happen around this country right now. Eight states and the District of Columbia have moved to legalize marijuana . . . these states are seeing decreases in violent crime," Booker said. "They're seeing their police forces be able to focus their time, energy, and resources [on] serious crime."

Booker was wrong. Completely.

When he made his announcement, only

four states — Alaska, Colorado, Oregon, Washington — had allowed recreational cannabis sales for more than a few months. (Voters in the District of Columbia and four others had also approved legalization at the time, but of that later group, only Nevada was allowing recreational sales, and it had just begun.)

So decent data on crime trends was — and is — available only on those first four states. Colorado and Washington are the largest of the four and were the first two to allow recreational sales, in 2014. Their last pre-legalization year was 2013. (Alaska and Oregon legalized in 2015, but for the sake of simplicity, I'll use 2013 data for them, too.)

State agencies like the Colorado Bureau of Investigation take a few months to compile data from local agencies, so the most recent statewide data available only covers 2017. Comparing 2017 to 2013 might seem like a fool's game — four years is hardly enough time to detect a trend either way.

Except it is. And the trend is ugly.

In 2013, Washington had 160 murders and about 11,700 aggravated assaults, according to statewide data that the Washington Association of Sheriffs & Police Chiefs provides to the FBI for its annual national crime report. In 2017, the state had 230 murders and 13,700 aggravated assaults — an increase of about 44 percent for murders and 17 percent for aggravated assaults. That increase far outpaced the national rise in crime. Murders rose about 20 percent nationally from 2013 to 2017, and aggravated assaults about 10 percent.

The other three states saw the same trend. In each of them, murders and serious assaults rose faster than the national average, even after accounting for population growth. Combined, the four states had about 450 murders and 30,300 aggravated assaults in 2013. They had about 615 murders and 37,800 aggravated assaults in 2017.

A statistical analysis showed only a 6 percent probability that the fact murders rose faster in the four marijuana states than the United States was due to chance — and almost no probability that the aggravated assault rise was due to chance.

The crime increase isn't a statistical anomaly. It's real.

Without examining each case, knowing how many crimes were marijuana related is impossible. But at the least, marijuana advocates need to stop claiming that legalization reduces violent crime when it so clearly doesn't.

Booker is fortunate that he's a media darling. A less-liked politician would have been called a liar for getting his facts so wrong.

But only if anyone knew the facts about marijuana and violence.

We live in an age of big data, an age when every news blip is tweeted instantly to millions. After a while, I began to wonder what I suspect you're wondering now: How could no one else know about these numbers? How could a senator make a false argument about marijuana and violence — while introducing a bill to legalize the drug nationally — without being called on his error?

How could the executive director of the Washington sheriffs' and police chiefs' association tell a newspaper in July 2017 that "it would be a strain to correlate violent crime and marijuana usage . . . I would struggle to believe that the legalization of marijuana or more legalization relates to violent crime"? Didn't he read his own group's report?

But modern policing in the United States is complicated. The Black Lives Matter movement has become a huge issue. So has the debate around firearm violence, and the question of the proper police response to the opioid epidemic.

Further, murder is extraordinarily rare, even in the United States. In 2013, the recent trough for crime, the risk that an American would be murdered had fallen to about 1-in-25,000. The risk that someone will commit murder is even lower, since some people kill more than once. Even in big, high-crime cities, the drivers of violence can take years to become obvious.

But there's another factor. Like everyone else, police officers face what scientists call confirmation bias. That term is a fancy way of saying that we look for evidence that supports what we think we already know. Cops see the connection between drugs and violence more intimately than anyone. But in Western states they often focus on the terrible crimes associated with methamphetamine. In big Eastern and Midwestern cities they look at heroin and cocaine dealing as a source of problems.

Like everyone else, they have been told for a generation that marijuana doesn't cause violence, that the belief it did came out of racist propaganda. The evidence to the contrary lies in dozens of different scientific journals and crime reports; it piles up month by month, but it's so scattered that almost no one has put it together.

Yet.

I grew to take a certain cold comfort in the PDFs filling folders on my computer. The studies and reports were real, even if no one knew about them. Besides, they were easier to read than the arrest warrants and news stories and police reports. I found victims even when I wasn't looking:

- Christian Pearson, 10, an Arizona boy allegedly beaten and burned to death by his mother and stepfather in June 2017. His mother told police officers she had just come home from a medical marijuana dispensary when she found him severely injured.
- Giovanni Diaz, 15, a Florida teen allegedly beaten to death with a baseball bat by his 16-year-old "best friend" in March 2018 after they smoked marijuana in a park.
- Jimi Patrick, 19, Dean Finocchiaro, 19, Thomas Meo, 21, and Mark Sturgis, 22, Pennsylvania men lured to a farm in July 2017 by a man who offered to sell them marijuana. Once they arrived, the dealer, who had been diagnosed with schizophrenia, killed them, burned three of their bodies, and buried all four in a mass grave.

- Mia Ayliffe-Chung, 20, and Tom Jackson, 30, British backpackers stabbed to death at a hostel in Queensland, Australia, in August 2016 by a French traveler. Judge Jean Dalton — the same judge who oversaw the Raina Thaiday child-killing case — found the killer not guilty by reason of marijuana-caused schizophrenia. He had smoked four cigarettes a day for years and believed the people at the hostel wanted to kill and cook him.
- Ashley Mead, 24, a Colorado mother killed by the father of her 1-year-old daughter in February 2017. He dismembered her body and left her torso in a Dumpster. In an arrest warrant, the Boulder police noted a large box "half-full of empty marijuana bottles" in the apartment Mead and her boyfriend shared and reported a neighbor smelled marijuana smoke constantly.
- The nineteen residents — yes, nineteen — at a Japanese nursing home stabbed to death in July 2016 by a 26-year-old man who had been hospitalized less than five months earlier for cannabis psychosis. Twenty-six other residents were wounded. According to a Japanese newspaper, the man told investi-

gators he wanted to legalize marijuana and believed drug gangs were targeting him, so he had no choice but to "complete his mission."

Do you want more cases? Because, unfortunately, there are plenty. The black tide of psychosis and the red tide of violence are rising together on a green wave, slow and steady and certain.

All anyone needs to do is look.

EPILOGUE:
WHAT NOW?

This book could have been longer.

The mental-health dangers of cannabis don't stop with psychosis. At a time when the suicide rate in the United States is rising, growing evidence links cannabis to depression and suicide. The Dunedin research also suggests that marijuana may lower overall intelligence, though other studies disagree with that finding.

A strong link between cannabis and dangerous driving is also emerging. The number of drivers in fatal accidents in Colorado and Washington who test positive for marijuana has soared since legalization. As with the marijuana-violence link, controlled laboratory research doesn't seem to capture the true risk.

An even broader question is whether persistent cannabis use decreases motivation and ultimately discourages users from working and having successful lives. Wayne

Hall, the Australian drug abuse expert, is hardly a cannabis alarmist. He notes that alcohol is far more physically toxic. Yet marijuana can subtly enmesh itself in the lives of users in ways that alcohol does not, he notes.

Those heavy users tend to be at a societal disadvantage already, and cannabis worsens it. Hall points to a New Zealand study — not Dunedin — that showed that people who used heavily into their late twenties generally had not married or found steady work. "They just didn't have much of a life, basically," Hall said. "That's one of the concerns that I would have about the social equity effects of legalization."

All these issues are important. But to me, at least, they are all secondary to marijuana's link to psychosis and violence — because the evidence is so strong, the issue so misunderstood, and the consequences so severe.

Now the time for guesswork is over. The federal government needs to step up with serious and well-funded research on marijuana's effects. Not on psychosis. That debate is over. By any reasonable standard, the connection has been proven.

But we need to know about the relationship between marijuana and other drug use.

The advocacy community made a brilliant tactical move when it promoted marijuana as a solution for the opiate crisis. In the very unlikely event marijuana can help people avoid opiate addiction, we should know, so we can encourage its use.

And in the far more likely event that marijuana is in fact a gateway drug, we should know — so that we don't push people who are at high risk for opiate addiction to use it.

We also need much more research into the marijuana-violence connection, to discover if marijuana causes as much violence as its link to psychosis and the emerging data suggests.

At the same time, the government should drop its barriers to researching cannabis for medical purposes. The reason is not that marijuana is likely to prove a miracle cure for cancer — or anything else. It's precisely the opposite. Let's put unfounded claims to rest, permanently.

If and when we do, I hope media outlets will pay as much attention to the negative findings as they have to the very slim positive ones so far. Journalists need to be far more skeptical when they discuss cannabis — both its risks and its potential benefits.

Marijuana is not medicine. Marijuana and

THC-extract products — whether eaten or smoked — are intoxicants and mild pain relievers, like alcohol. They have serious side effects, like alcohol. Serious journalists don't pretend alcohol is medicine. They need to stop extending that false courtesy to marijuana.

(Yes, CBD is medicine, in the traditional sense. It has won FDA approval to treat a medical condition. But CBD is not marijuana. It is a single chemical compound derived from marijuana. It has less to do with cannabis than morphine has to do with the poppy plant. Morphine effectively concentrates the natural ability of poppy flowers to produce pain relief and euphoria, while CBD has none of the psychoactive properties that cause people to use marijuana and THC recreationally.)

Further, the civil rights issues around marijuana legalization are far more complicated than the media or politicians would like them to be. Yes, marijuana arrests disproportionately fall on minorities, especially the black community.

But marijuana's harms also disproportionately fall on the black community. Black people are more likely to develop cannabis use disorder. They are also more likely to develop schizophrenia — and much more likely to be perpetrators and victims of violence. Given marijuana's connection with mental illness and violence, it is reasonable to wonder whether the drug is partly responsible for those differentials.

In general, the reporting around marijuana and legalization has been ridiculously lopsided. The media owes us all a more thoughtful understanding of the risks and benefits.

Time is running short.

Even as I write this book, the evidence that cannabis causes mental illness and violence is becoming stronger. New studies and new data have emerged. And yet even as I wrote this book, marijuana's move toward legalization in the United States gained momentum. In a single week in June 2018, voters in Oklahoma approved medical marijuana, Charles Schumer, a US senator from New York, introduced federal decriminalization legislation, and Canada became the second country to legalize marijuana fully. (The first, Uruguay, began retail sales in the fall of 2017; in the first six months of 2018, murders in Uruguay rose 64 percent compared to the same period in 2017. Coincidence, no doubt.)

Eventually these two trends must collide.

But how many people will become psychotic or violent before politicians and the advocacy community admit the risks of legalization? And full legalization will draw billions of dollars in new investment into cannabis businesses, making restrictions even more difficult.

When I told people I was writing this book, they inevitably asked whether I thought marijuana should be legal. Like Robin Murray, I usually dodged the question. Legalization appeared certain, and I simply wanted people to understand the risks, I said.

But the truth is: No. Of course, it shouldn't.

The best reason to legalize marijuana is not a good one. It's that alcohol is legal, and alcohol is responsible for significant violence and death. But alcohol is far more ingrained in American society than marijuana. Criminalizing it would be impossible, as Prohibition proved. Over half of Americans have had a drink in the last month.

Despite what its backers claim, marijuana is still a relatively marginal drug. Half of Americans have never used it. More than 85 percent have not done so in the past year. As you've seen, its consumption is concentrated among a vocal minority of heavy users.

Alcohol is certainly more physically harmful than marijuana, but marijuana is more neurotoxic. Alcohol rarely causes psychosis except in late-stage drinkers. And the kind of violence that alcohol causes is very different — and, yes, less severe — than the violence that marijuana causes.

There are no victims, cops sometimes say. What they mean is that violence victims are rarely completely innocent. The person who winds up dead after a bar fight or a gang shooting might easily have been the killer.

But marijuana's madness makes its victims exceptions. They are children, wives, parents, even strangers, people whose only crime was being near someone in the grip of psychosis. That risk — not racism — is the reason that societies have always been wary of marijuana. And the new high-THC products worsen it. Why on earth would we want to encourage people to use this drug?

The direct economic benefits of legalization also appear to be vastly overstated. In the first states to legalize, sales are already peaking. In May 2018, Colorado quietly hit a milestone that the cannabis industry didn't publicize. For the first time, overall year-over-year retail sales fell. Counting medical and recreational dispensaries, marijuana sales were $122.9 million, compared to $123.5 million in May 2017. (Overall consumption probably is still rising slightly, but because of oversupply, prices are falling.)

Colorado's retail market is about $1.5 billion, and the state collected about $250 million in taxes in 2017 — both rounding errors compared to the state's overall economy of $300 billion and budget of $29 billion. Considering that hospitalizing a patient with psychosis for a single ten-day inpatient stay costs more than $10,000 — and that few of those patients have private insurance — it is possible that the costs of marijuana psychosis and violence alone already outweigh the taxes the industry pays in Colorado. (That comparison takes no account of any other costs associated with marijuana.)

Decriminalization is a reasonable compromise. People shouldn't be arrested or sent to jail for possessing marijuana. If they're dumb enough to smoke in public, the police should take their joints and ticket them. If they're dumb enough to be caught smoking while they're on parole, they should be sent back to prison. But if they want to use in the privacy of their own homes, so be it.

But legalization is very different, which is exactly why marijuana's backers are pushing so hard for it. Legalization creates an entrenched business community that can promote its product. Legalization encourages investment and drives down the price of cannabis. In states that haven't legalized, an ounce of pot usually costs in the range of $300 — as much as six times the price in states like Oregon. (And as you've seen, the home cultivation allowed under legalization feeds a black market with even lower prices.)

Most of all, legalization signals that marijuana is not dangerous and encourages teen use. The states with the highest rates of youth marijuana use all allow legalized recreational sales or medical sales with very loose conditions.

The United States should not legalize cannabis nationally; it should move to discourage more states from legalizing, and it should consider pressuring those that have already done so to reverse course. Theoretically middle-ground alternatives to reduce the risk of legalized cannabis, such as regulating its THC content or imposing high taxes, won't work in practice. They will simply lead to a black market in potent, untaxed marijuana.

But Robin Murray is right that the precise legal status of marijuana is less important than public understanding of the risks. Most people who smoke cigarettes don't die of lung cancer, but we say that cigarettes cause cancer, full stop. We make sure anyone who smokes knows the risk. Most people who drink and drive don't have accidents, but we highlight the cases of those who do. Most people who smoke marijuana will not develop psychosis or commit violence, but we need to make sure that everyone who smokes knows the reality of the connection.

Only adults — preferably over 25 — should use cannabis. And they should use only if they are psychiatrically healthy. Instead, at the moment, cannabis advocates are encouraging the most dangerous type of use — long-term use of THC as an antidepressant or antianxiety drug, by people as young as 18, whose brains are still developing.

And so we are in the worst of all possible worlds. Marijuana is legal in some states, illegal in others, becoming steadily more potent, and sold without warnings everywhere. We have nearly ended youth cigarette smoking with pointed, well-funded advertising campaigns. Between 2002 and 2014, the rate of tobacco use among adolescents fell from 13 percent to under 5 percent. Teens are now more likely to use cannabis than cigarettes.

If we do nothing else, we need to commit to discouraging young people from using marijuana just as we do with tobacco. The personal and societal costs of psychosis are just too high.

Twenty years ago, the United States moved to allow or encourage wider use of two drugs: cannabis and opiates. In both cases, we ignored hundreds of years of warnings. We decided that we knew better, that we could outsmart the drug and somehow have its benefits without its costs.

We were wrong. Opiates are far riskier, of course, and the overdose deaths they cause more obvious, and so we have focused on those. But soon enough the mental illness and violence that marijuana use causes will be too widespread to ignore.

Writing this book was a depressing exercise, as you might imagine. Every day I read about marijuana, violence, and psychosis — and every day I read the cheery tales told by cannabis advocates. But when I got too down, I reminded myself that the situation now isn't unlike the late 1970s, the last time that cannabis was so widely used in the United States.

Then, like now, many advocates believed that the United States was moving inevitably toward legalization. In the 1970s, more teenagers were using, so more parents could see marijuana's negative effects firsthand — but, on the other hand, the drug was far less potent, so its neurotoxicity wasn't so obvious. And in the late 1970s, once enough people experienced marijuana's impacts up close, the tide shifted almost instantly.

Even now, despite the daily bombardment of pro-cannabis messages, hints that marijuana's popularity may be peaking are emerging. Alongside the Colorado sales peak and the Oregon supply glut, sales in California in 2018 are falling short of industry forecasts. A drug that regularly causes paranoia and psychosis may be less appealing than its backers think.

And a non-governmental lobbying group is now fighting cannabis legalization nationally. In 2013, Kevin Sabet, a former advisor in the Office of National Drug Control Policy, founded Smart Approaches to Marijuana to advocate for policies to discourage use of the drug. The pro-legalization groups still dwarf it in size and influence, but SAM has grown to a $2 million annual budget — with no money coming from opioid, alcohol, or tobacco companies — and affiliates in almost every state.

Still, I am old enough to understand how

difficult a task I have set myself with this book. If you are an average American, you believe both medical and recreational marijuana should be legal. I'm trying to change your mind. And changing someone's mind is next to impossible. I mean anyone's mind, of anything. People think what they think. So, this book all by itself may not do much.

But I hope at the least it will make you skeptical of the pro-marijuana arguments that advocates have sold you for twenty-five years. More, I hope it will open your eyes to the mental illness and violence that marijuana causes in your community, whether that community is Bellingham or Burlington, Five Points in Denver or Little Five Points in Atlanta, Park Slope or Pacific Heights. Nothing is more powerful than personal experience.

Open your eyes.

See the truth.

Tell your children.

ACKNOWLEDGMENTS

I've spent the last several years writing novels, a solitary process, at times desperately so. A work of nonfiction is far different. In writing this book I asked many people for help, and most were generous with their time and knowledge. They included everyone from people with schizophrenia to scientists on four continents. I didn't have space to quote them all in this book, but they were all helpful.

Psychiatrists, researchers, and scientists who shared their knowledge — in person, over the phone, or via email — included:

Seth Ammerman, Sven Andréasson, Louise Arseneault, Jacob Ballon, Sagnik Bhattacharyya, Mary Cannon, Marta Di Forti, Cyril D'Souza, Amir Englund, Seena Fazel, Tom Freeman, Wayne Hall, Julie Gazmararian, Robert Heinssen, Kevin Heslin, Shelaigh Hodgins, John Huffman, James Kirkbride, Emily Kline, Matthew Large, Bernard

Le Foll, Valentina Lorenzetti, Michael Lynskey, Erik Messamore, Nathaniel Morris, Valerie Moulin, Robin Murray, Olav Nielssen, Mark Olfson, Elyse Phillips, Aneta Lotakov Prince, Genie Roosevelt, Russell Russo, Melanie Rylander, Phil Silva, Scott Simpson, Christian Thurstone, Jim van Os, Nora Volkow, Cathy Wasserman, and George Wang. If anyone has slipped my mind, I apologize.

Any and all errors are mine and mine alone. Sometimes that sentence is boilerplate, but in this case, it couldn't be truer. The science around psychosis is complicated. I have done my best to explain accurately what the experts say, but the mistakes belong to me.

I drew on histories and memoirs from Patrick Anderson, Bruce Barcott, Isaac Campos, Emily Dufton, John Hudak, Michael Massing, Martin Torgoff — and of course George Francis William Ewens. I do wonder what Ewens would make of the modern American marijuana industry, with its budtenders and delivery apps. *Marijuana: What Everyone Needs to Know,* by Jonathan P. Caulkins, Beau Kilmer, and Mark A. R. Kleiman, offered a balanced look at the pros and cons of legalization (though it understates the violence risk).

The Institute of Medicine/National Academy of Medicine reports from 1999 and 2017 were comprehensive, thoughtful — and showed how scientific knowledge of the risks of marijuana has risen even as popular and political views have swung the other way.

Ethan Nadelmann, Marcia Rosenbaum, and Rob Kampia were generous with their time. So was Marcus Bachhuber, the author of the 2014 *JAMA Internal Medicine* paper.

In Colorado, the 18th Judicial District Attorney's Office provided the investigative file on the Kevin Lyons case at no cost and made district attorney George Brauchler, Darcy Kofol, and other senior attorneys available for an interview. Medical examiners' offices in several counties provided autopsy reports, usually at no charge.

Richard Kirk offered me his version of his life and the night of April 14, 2014; his in-laws Marti and Wayne Kohnke spoke candidly about an extraordinarily painful event. So did Kirk's friend Patrick Milligan. David Rosen, Kirk's lawyer, helped put me in touch with him, and Tina Fraker and others at the Bent County Correctional Facility courteously arranged my visit.

Danielle Caho fearlessly recounted how her boyfriend Christopher Pepper and his mother Barbara were shot in Colorado Springs by Elijah Tyre Colon in May 2017 as she was in another room. (Days before she was murdered, Barb had asked Danielle and her son not to smoke marijuana with Colon. She said she didn't like the way the drug made Colon act. But I couldn't be certain Colon had used on the evening he killed the Peppers, so I did not include the murder in the main body of the book. Colon pled guilty in 2018 and is now serving a seventy-year sentence.) Michael Allen, who prosecuted Colon, also took time to talk about the case with me.

Susan Riehl told me about her son Matthew, and Sheridan Orr about her brother Kevin. Eric and his family gave me a glimpse inside their lives.

Any number of people with psychosis told me about their own struggles, but aside from David Louis Bragen, who is named in the book, I'm protecting their privacy.

Almost sixteen years ago, Jon Karp published my first nonfiction book. Jon, thanks for taking a chance on me again, on an even more controversial topic. Mitchell Ivers told me to follow the facts, wherever they led. Natasha Simons and Hannah Brown saw the manuscript over the finish line. Robert Barnett and Deneen Howell offered advice and counsel.

Peter Bach, my brother David, and Andrew Ross Sorkin all read a first draft and made thoughtful comments.

A special thanks to Sanford Gordon, who took time out from his own work to do mine. I owe you, Sandy.

And, finally — this book would not have been possible without my wife, Dr. Jacqueline Berenson. And I don't mean that in the usual pro forma "This wouldn't have been possible without my spouse" way. Jackie's work as a forensic psychiatrist gives her a unique perspective on the violence that marijuana causes. Her understanding of the issue led me down the path to this book.

I hope I've done it — and her — justice.

ABOUT THE AUTHOR

Alex Berenson is a former *New York Times* reporter and award-winning novelist. Born in New York, he attended Yale University and went on to join the *New York Times* in 1999. There he covered everything from the drug industry to Hurricane Katrina and served two stints as a correspondent in Iraq. His time in Iraq led him to write *The Faithful Spy,* his debut novel, which won the Edgar Award for Best First Novel from the Mystery Writers of America. Currently, he lives in the Hudson Valley with his wife and children, writes fiction, and still occasionally contributes to the *Times* and other publications. *Tell Your Children* is his second nonfiction book.

The employees of Thorndike Press hope you have enjoyed this Large Print book. All our Thorndike, Wheeler, and Kennebec Large Print titles are designed for easy reading, and all our books are made to last. Other Thorndike Press Large Print books are available at your library, through selected bookstores, or directly from us.

For information about titles, please call:
(800) 223-1244

or visit our website at:
gale.com/thorndike

To share your comments, please write:
Publisher
Thorndike Press
10 Water St., Suite 310
Waterville, ME 04901